THE COMPLETE GUIDE TO

POSTNATAL FITNESS

Other Titles in THE **COMPLETE GUIDES** SERIES

The Complete Guide to
Circuit Training
by Debbie Lawrence, Bob Hope

The Complete Guide to
Core Stability
by Matt Lawrence

The Complete Guide to
Endurance Training
by Jon Ackland

The Complete Guide to
Strength Training
2nd edition
by Anita Bean

The Complete Guide to
Exercise in Water
by Debbie Lawrence

The Complete Guide to
Stretching
by Christopher Norris

The Complete Guide to
Exercise to Music
2nd edition
by Debbie Lawrence

The Complete Guide to
Sports Massage
by Tim Paine

THE **COMPLETE GUIDE TO**

Judy DiFiore

POSTNATAL
FITNESS

2nd edition

A & C Black • London

Second edition published in 2003
by A & C Black (Publishers) Ltd
37 Soho Square, London W1D 3QZ

First edition 1998

ISBN 0 7136 6454 1

A CIP catalogue record for this book is available from the British Library.

Acknowledgements
Cover photograph copyright © Mother & Baby Picture Library/Dave Anthony.
Illustrations by Jean Ashley.

A & C Black uses paper produced with elemental chlorine-free pulp, harvested from managed sustainable forests.

Typeset in 10½ on 12pt Baskerville BE Regular

Printed and bound in Great Britain by

CONTENTS

ACKNOWLEDGEMENTS

Whilst this edition has been completely revised I still owe gratitude to those involved with the original version. I would like to thank YMCA Fitness Industry Training for giving me the opportunity to deliver and develop the ante/postnatal teacher training module for 14 years and for providing a platform for recognition. A special mention to the three physiotherapists originally involved with this course, Molly Jennings, Sue Lewis and Gillian Fletcher, whose enthusiasm and dedication to ante- and postnatal exercise inspired me to work in this field 14 years ago.

For this edition I would like to thank Samantha Gillard, Clinical Specialist in Women's Health Physiotheraphy for editing the pelvic floor chapter and dear friend Sue Lewis, Chartered Physiotherapist in Women's Health for proof-reading Part 1. I would also like to thank them both for their assistance with the numerous queries that arose.

Thanks also to two very special friends and colleagues: Tricia Liggett for her inspirational work on alignment and for introducing me to the delights of the foam roller and Jenny Tarsnane for reviewing the exercise sections.

I could not have written this without the hands-on experience of real postnatal teaching, so I would like to thank all my postnatal mums and their babies, over the last 14 years, for helping me learn and develop from them and for making my job so rewarding.

Above all, I would like to thank my wonderful husband Mike for supporting me, whilst I juggled full-time teaching commitments and family life with writing this book!

INTRODUCTION

Many women are anxious to get themselves back into shape as soon as possible after baby is born. Although her body may not resemble its former shape, a woman will feel relieved that it is her own again and can move freely in a more co-ordinated, unrestricted way. Inspired by a wobbly abdomen and leaky breasts and pelvic floor, she needs sound guidance and understanding to help her along the road to recovery and fitness. It isn't just a matter of starting where she left off and resuming her pre-pregnancy programme; pregnancy and delivery have implications for her exercising body which she should be aware of before she begins. Consider the key postnatal issues of reduced joint stability, stretched and weakened pelvic floor and abdominal muscles, and large, heavy breasts, to understand that the body is really quite vulnerable at this time.

For the purpose of health-related fitness it is recommended that women do not commence formal exercise until completion of a satisfactory postnatal check-up. We hear of elite athletes who return to training within two weeks of delivery because they want to capitalise on physiological changes that have occurred during pregnancy. This is all very well in the pursuit of athletic success, but there are risks involved which are certainly not worth taking if health-related fitness is the goal. Return to fitness and regular weight should be viewed as a long-term goal which cannot be achieved in a short space of time.

About the guide

The Complete Guide to Postnatal Fitness was written in response to the demand for more detailed information on the subject from group fitness instructors and personal trainers. It goes a step further than other postnatal exercise books and looks at specific training methods, their suitability, and considerations during the postnatal period. Research in this field of exercise is continually improving and, where available, resultant information has been cited, but there are some areas which lack any scientific evidence at all. In such cases, I have based my recommendations on sound knowledge of the anatomical and physiological implications of pregnancy and delivery, together with many years experience of teaching postnatal women.

How to use the guide

Whilst it is hoped you will read the guide from cover to cover, it is also intended as an essential resource for you to dip in and out of as required. With this in mind, the chapters are all self-contained and cross-referenced as necessary.

- Part One looks at the implications of pregnancy and delivery in detail, in particular how these will affect the return to exercise in the postnatal period, and how it can help the body to recover more quickly.

- Part Two is all about exercise. It looks at core stability, cardiovascular and resistance training methods, and a range of group exercise sessions, for their suitability during the postnatal period.
- Part Three is concerned with planning and teaching a specific postnatal exercise session and the strategies involved in its success.

For ease of writing, baby is referred to as 'he' in the text; the early postnatal period is defined as birth to six weeks; the extended postnatal period is anything after that time.

Benefits of postnatal exercise

Posture

- Correction of pregnancy stance.
- Improved core strength.
- Strengthened muscles that have lengthened.
- Lengthened muscles that have shortened.
- Redressed muscular balance.
- Awareness of posture whilst feeding/lifting/carrying.
- Awareness of back, abdominal and pelvic care.

Functional capacity

- Targeting muscles required for baby care.
- Increased strength and endurance for lifting, carrying and performing one-handed tasks.
- Improved core strength.
- Improved aerobic fitness.
- Increased ability to deal with the everyday demands of a new baby.
- Reduced fatigue – increased energy.

General health

- Boosted immune system.
- Improved sleep quality.
- Improved circulation and healing.
- Improved digestion.

Body composition

- Increased muscle mass.
- Increased metabolic rate.
- Increased caloric burning.
- Increased fat loss.

Social and emotional well-being

- Increased production of endorphins.
- Enhanced self image and self-confidence.
- Personal satisfaction.
- Personal identification.
- Increased social interaction.

Risks of postnatal exercise

- Fatigue and exhaustion.
- Injury from reduced joint stability.
- Injury from poor core stability.
- Injury from inappropriate exercises or technique.
- Reduction in milk quality and production.

Contra-indications to exercise

- Joint or pelvic pain.
- Inadequate healing, discomfort.
- Excessive fatigue.
- Gross divarication of rectus abdominis.

THE IMPLICATIONS OF PREGNANCY AND DELIVERY FOR EXERCISE

PART ONE

STRUCTURE AND ALIGNMENT

The Spine

Structure of the spine

Fig. 1.1	Structure of the spine

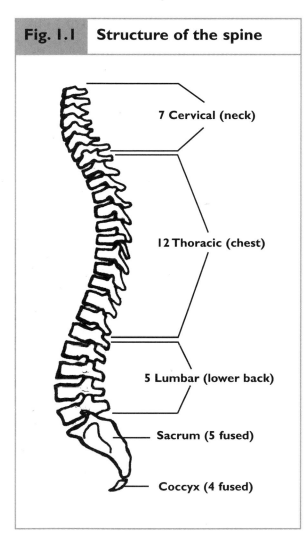

7 Cervical (neck)

12 Thoracic (chest)

5 Lumbar (lower back)

Sacrum (5 fused)

Coccyx (4 fused)

The vertebral column is made up of 33 bones: 24 separate vertebrae, five vertebrae fused together to form the sacrum, and another four vertebrae fused together to form the coccyx. The spine has enormous strength, but since it is made up of small sections it is also very flexible and this allows a large range of movement. The vertebrae are separated by intervertebral discs of fibrocartilage that cushion the vertebrae against jarring and help to keep the spine upright. The curves of the spine are vital for shock absorption; without them the base of the brain would receive the full impact when jumping. The spine is dependent on ligaments as well as muscles for its stability.

Effects of pregnancy on the spine

The stability of the spine is seriously at risk during pregnancy for the following reasons.

- Increased elasticity of the ligaments.
- Forward pull of the abdomen as the uterus grows out of the pelvis into the abdominal cavity.
- Increased load, causing the sacrum to tilt downwards and forwards.
- Over-stretched abdominal muscles which are no longer able to support the spine.
- Increased size and weight of the breasts.

Common changes in spinal alignment result in increased lumbar lordosis, thoracic kyphosis and cervical lordosis as a consequence of the latter.

Fig. 1.2	Effects of pregnancy on the spine

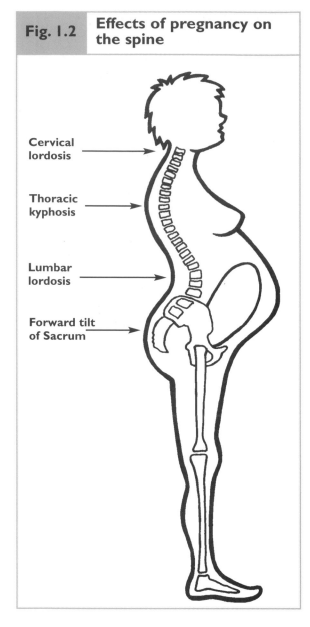

Cervical lordosis

Thoracic kyphosis

Lumbar lordosis

Forward tilt of Sacrum

The pelvis

The bones of the pelvis

The pelvis is made up of four bones: two hip bones, the sacrum and the coccyx. Each hip bone is made up of three fused bones, the ilium, ischium and pubis. At the junction of these three bones is the deep socket of the acetabulum.

- The **ilium** is the large wing-shaped part of the pelvis providing a broad surface area for muscle attachment. The upper border, the iliac crest, can be felt when the hands are placed on the hips. The bony points at each end of the iliac crest can be felt at the front, as the anterior superior iliac spines (ASIS) and at the back, as the posterior superior iliac spines (PSIS) of the pelvis. These are useful landmarks when checking correct postural alignment.
- The **ischium** is the thick, lower part of the pelvis leading down to the ischial tuberosities.
- The **pubis** is at the front of the pelvis where the two pubic bones join to form the symphysis pubis at the top and the pubic arch underneath.
- The **sacrum** is a triangular-shaped bone made up of five fused vertebrae. It is joined to the ilium by the sacroiliac joints, which are positioned on either side of the sacrum.

Fig. 1.3	Bones of the pelvis

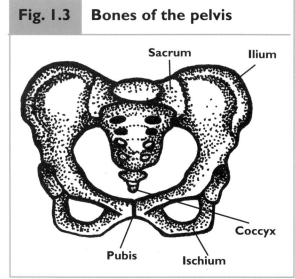

Sacrum

Ilium

Coccyx

Pubis

Ischium

- The **coccyx** consists of four fused vertebrae joined to the sacrum at the sacrococcygeal joint. This joint has a small amount of movement that may allow the coccyx to be pushed backwards during delivery.

Fig. 1.4	Joints of pelvis showing ligaments

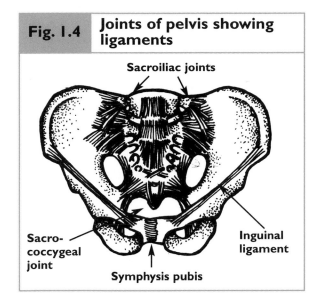

The joints of the pelvis

The pelvis is formed by two halves that join at the front at the symphysis pubis and at the back at the sacroiliac joints.

- Symphysis pubis is situated at the front of the pelvis, where the two pubic bones meet. Separated by a pad of cartilage resembling a vertebral disc, the joint is approximately 4mm wide prior to pregnancy and held together by ligaments.
- Sacroiliac joints are two joints formed by the unity of the ilium with the sacrum at each side. The strongest joints in the body, they are held together by ligaments. They allow very limited backwards and forwards movement during flexion and extension of the trunk (sacral nodding) as well as a sideways tilt which occurs when walking.

Effects of pregnancy on the pelvis

The three joints of the pelvis – one symphysis pubis and two sacroiliac – are vulnerable during pregnancy. Hormonal changes allow the ligaments supporting these three joints to become more elastic, increasing their range of movement and consequently reducing joint stability. The width of the symphysis pubis may increase to 9 mm, causing severe discomfort around the pubis and groin, and in severe cases the joint may separate. In some cases however, pain around the pubis may not always be reflective of the degree of movement at the joint. This condition is known as symphysis pubis dysfunction (*see* section on symphysis pubis pain on page 49). Increased laxity in the sacroiliac joints may cause pain in one or both sides of the pelvis. Alternatively, pain could be the result of the two joint surfaces becoming stuck together, causing stiffness and reduced mobility.

The pelvis is dependent upon the correct alignment of the symphysis pubis and sacroiliac joints and pain experienced in one area is generally consistent with misalignment of the whole structure.

Relaxin

What is relaxin?

Research has identified relaxin as a hormone produced in both pregnant and non-pregnant women (Bani 1997). Produced primarily by the corpus luteum, it reaches its highest levels during pregnancy when it is also produced by the placenta and the decidua. Increased levels of relaxin are evident in the body from as early as the second week of pregnancy and continue until delivery. Monthly production resumes with the recommencement of the menstrual cycle. Relaxin levels are higher in second and subsequent pregnancies and in women carrying more than one baby.

What effects do increased levels of relaxin have on the body during pregnancy?

The most significant change occurs in the collagen fibres of connective tissue, found in cartilage, tendons, ligaments, muscles, skin etc. Increased levels of relaxin appear to affect the remodelling structure of collagen fibres by increasing the water content which in turn increases their size and elasticity. This directly affects joint stability as the ligaments are unable to provide the same degree of support as before.

Increased elasticity of the ligaments allows the pelvic joints a greater range of movement and, together with the forward tilt of the sacrum, increases the size of the pelvic outlet by 28 per cent. This is vital to accommodate the growing baby and allow an easier birth.

Which joints are most at risk?

All joints will be affected to some degree and although there is concern for the ankles, knees and elbows during exercise, it is the pelvic joints that are mostly at risk. The symphysis pubis and sacroiliac joints are cartilaginous, or slightly moveable, joints that rely solely on ligaments for their stability. The resulting increased range of movement created by relaxin, together with the progressive pressure exerted by the growing baby, makes these joints particularly vulnerable.

Are muscles affected by relaxin?

Connective tissue surrounds bundles of muscle fibres that merge together and extend beyond the muscle to form the tough, inelastic tendon. The relaxing effects of the collagenous fibres afford a greater range of movement for the muscle and its attachments. It is essential for the abdominal muscles to stretch to allow the uterus to grow out of the abdomen, and for the pelvic floor muscles to stretch to deliver the baby. However, this adaptation severely reduces the support previously given by these muscles and has major implications on muscle function and support (*see* Chapters 2 and 3).

What happens to relaxin after delivery?

Production of relaxin ceases on delivery of the placenta. However, the changes that have occurred to the collagen fibres will continue until new tissue has been reformed in the absence of relaxin. This may be a period of up to five months postnatally. Reduced joint stability should still be strongly considered when exercising postnatally as the body continues to be vulnerable during this time.

Do the joints regain their stability?

If the joints have been overextended during pregnancy, the ligaments may not provide sufficient stabilisation. However, if appropriate care has been taken the ligaments should return to their pre-pregnancy inelastic state once the lingering effects of relaxin have left the body. The absence of pressure from the baby greatly reduces the risks to the pelvis, but whilst the increased range of movement is still evident the pelvis should be treated with much respect and caution.

Breastfeeding women may find increased joint laxity continues until feeding stops although there is no evidence to support this at present.

Posture

Posture is strongly influenced by habit and controlled by our own kinesthetic awareness, good or bad, of what 'feels right'. Correct postural alignment is governed by the strength and suppleness of specific muscles. Good posture is not a static position; correct alignment is constantly challenged as the body moves.

Why is correct posture so important?

When the body is misaligned it has to work harder to maintain an upright stance. Muscles that are not designed to support the body are recruited to take up the slack and they become too tight. In addition to placing extra strain on the joints and their support structures, tight muscles will decrease range of movement and pull the body out of alignment. If that's not enough, overly lax muscles tire easily in the attempt to counterbalance the forces and the body begins to sag. Such changes in muscular balance increase the degree of compression on the vertebrae and intervertebral discs and decrease blood flow.

Postnatal posture

The following biomechanical changes are the most commonly observed as a result of pregnancy.

Increased lumbar lordosis:
- Shortening and tightening of iliopsoas and lengthening and weakening of gluteus maximus occur as the sacrum, and sometimes the whole pelvis, tilts anteriorly.
- The facets of lumbar vertebrae become compressed so the hamstrings tighten to

Fig. 1.5	Musculoskeletal and biomechanical changes

Centre of gravity moves forward

Trapezius rhomboids lengthen

Pectorals tighten

Lower ribcage flares

Rectus abdominis lengthens

Transversus abdominis lengthens

Lumbar extensors tighten

Iliopsoas tightens

Gluteus maximus lengthens

Hamstrings tighten

draw down the ischial tuberosities in an attempt to protect the spine.
- The hamstrings become overactive and tight as they hang on to the tilting pelvis.

5

- Lumbar extensors shorten and tighten whilst transversus abdominis weakens.
- Rectus abdominis lengthens, weakens and possibly separates.
- Poor functional use of the abdominal wall reduces stability in the pelvis and lower back.

Thoracic kyphosis:
- Shortening and tightening of pectoralis minor occurs with the increased size of the breasts which is further enhanced by poor feeding positions.
- Corresponding lengthening and weakening occurs in trapezius/rhomboids.
- The lower rib cage flares to accommodate the baby.
- Cervical lordosis increases with tilting of head forward.

Postural retraining is crucial to redress the balance of pregnancy-induced changes, and an awareness of correct alignment should be rigorously observed.

Key aims for restoring correct posture
- Re-establish good body alignment.
- Increase core stability.
- Balance opposing muscle groups through strength/stretch.

Correct spinal alignment

Neutral spine is the natural alignment of the spine, i.e. inward curve of the lumbar and cervical vertebrae and outward curve of the thoracic vertebrae. In this position, pressure is equally distributed along the length of the spine, enabling the back to absorb impact whilst minimising stress on bone and soft tissue. When the spine is balanced in neutral, body weight is supported primarily through the

bones. Only a very small amount of muscular contraction is needed, from the abdominals and spinal extensors, to maintain equilibrium.

Benefits of neutral spine include:

- Improved body mechanics and neuro-muscular efficiency
- Reduction and/or elimination of pain
- Prevention of injury
- Improved circulation
- Improved body shape and a more slender appearance
- Increased flexibility
- Improved co-ordination and sense of balance
- Release of pent-up tensions

Maintaining the spine in a neutral position is extremely difficult for many people. It is often misunderstood and performed incorrectly by over-tilting and eliminating the natural lumbar curve.

Finding neutral spine

Stand with feet hip-width apart and knees soft. Place the heel of your hands on the prominent bones at the front of your pelvis (ASIS) and fingertips on your pubic bone. Tilt the top of the pelvis forward so that your fingertips are lower than the heel of your hand and the natural curvature in your back has increased (anterior pelvic tilt). Now tilt your pelvis the opposite way by lifting your pubic bone upwards so that your fingertips are higher than the heel of your hand (posterior pelvic tilt). Feel your back straightening as the natural curvature disappears. Now find a position midway between these two extremes where your fingertips and heel of hands are on the same vertical plane. Buttocks and front of thighs should be relaxed. This is your correct spinal alignment also known as 'neutral spine'.

Fig. 1.6	Correct (left) and incorrect (right) posture

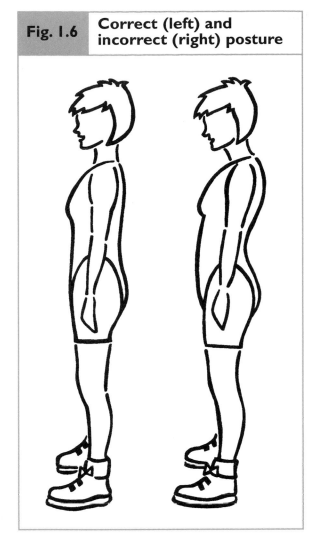

Standing posture
- Stand with the feet hip-width apart (underneath ASIS).
- Spread weight equally between both feet.
- Distribute weight evenly between big toe, little toe and heel.
- Soften the knees and align them over the ankles.
- Find your neutral spine (see above).
- Draw navel through to spine.

- Slide your shoulders down and open the chest.
- Lengthen your tailbone towards the floor.
- Extend your spine towards the ceiling.
- Lengthen the neck keeping the chin parallel to the floor.
- Look straight ahead.

Back care

A new baby makes many new and repetitive demands on the body. Getting in and out of bed for unsociable feeds, bending over to change nappies, securing car seats, and lifting and carrying baby and his accompanying equipment all require the body to work in a variety of physically demanding ways. The spine and pelvis can all too easily be twisted when lowering the car seat into position and securing the seat belt, and the spine can be badly stressed if the large muscles of the legs are not used for bending and lifting. Guidelines for safe practice can be found in the Appendix.

Relaxin and postnatal exercise

The lingering effects of relaxin on joint stability is one of the main risk factors of postnatal exercise. The following areas should be considered.

Range of movement
Care should be taken to protect the joints against injury by ensuring all movements are performed within the regular range of the joint. Speed becomes very important here as fast, particularly long-levered, movements will increase momentum and could easily result in overextension of the joint. Activities such as

Tai-bo, kick boxing, karate etc. may carry an additional risk as the fast, jerky, movements may encourage joint locking or twisting. Studio resistance classes should be avoided by inexperienced participants; skilled individuals may return to the activity once core strength has been regained. Range of movement should be considered with some yoga postures to avoid overextending unstable joints.

Alignment and technique

All movements should be performed with correct body alignment and attention to technical detail. Locking out, or hyperextension, of elbows and knees should be avoided at all times. Neutral spine should be maintained throughout and a tall upright stance adopted where appropriate. Movements involving repetitive joint actions, such as the stepper or cross-trainer, should be kept to a minimum and range adjusted to avoid misalignment of the pelvis. Gym and studio cycling may cause discomfort in symphysis pubis and/or sacroiliac joints if correct seat height is not established. Increased Q angle of the femur may cause knee misalignment during all weight-bearing activities.

Flexibility work

Stretching to increase flexibility should be avoided until 16–20 weeks after the baby is born, or longer if breastfeeding continues. Attempting to take a stretch further than the range of the joint permits could severely compromise joint stability, and the overextension of ligaments may be permanent. Stretching to *maintain* muscle length is strongly recommended and crucial for rebalancing posture. Comfortable stretch positions can be held for longer (up to 30 sec) but no attempt should be made to try and stretch further. Some yoga postures may encourage overextension particularly since they are often held for some time. Care should be taken when participating in this type of activity in the first few months after delivery and instructors should provide alternative postures where appropriate.

High-impact activities

These should also be avoided for the first few months to allow sufficient time for joint and pelvic floor recovery. Lactating breasts will feel uncomfortable and place further stress on their delicate support structures. Pressure on the joints is increased twofold with high-impact activities and puts particular strain on the ankles, knees, pelvis and spine. Jogging is only appropriate if a low-impact stride is practised, minimising vertical action and absorbing the shock through a heel–toe action. Correct knee–hip alignment should also be observed. Experienced runners may need to review their technique.

Resistance training

This relates to the use of resistance equipment in the gym or a studio resistance class. Experienced lifters who continued to train during pregnancy should recommence at the same resistance they were lifting prior to delivery. If resistance training was not undertaken during pregnancy they should recommence at 70 per cent of what they were lifting prior to pregnancy. A heavy weight pulling on an unstable joint has serious implications and should be avoided until the muscles and joints regain strength and stability. A further area of concern with the use of weights is the reduction in core strength and the resulting compromise in postural alignment. It is for this reason that it is not advisable for newcomers to exercise with weights – core abdominal strength must be established before adding resistance (*see* Chapter 8). Technical teaching is vital, with information about getting into and out of the machine as well as about the exercise itself. Close observation and correction by the instructor should be expected.

Summary

- Relaxin affects the collagen fibres of connective tissue.
- Joints continue to be at risk from the lingering effects of relaxin which caused increased elasticity of the ligaments during pregnancy.
- The effects may continue for up to five months after delivery.
- Joint laxity may persist for longer if breastfeeding.
- The sacroiliac and symphysis pubis joints of the pelvis are particularly vulnerable to injury.
- Posture must be retrained following pregnancy, and essential back care learnt during everyday baby care.
- Neutral spinal alignment should be constantly practised.
- All movements should be performed within the regular range of the joint.
- High-impact activities should be avoided for the first few months after delivery.
- Core stability should be increased before adding resistance.
- Resistance programmes should be endurance-based.
- Overextension of any joint must be avoided.
- Correct joint alignment and exercise technique is vital.
- Flexibility work should be avoided until 16–20 weeks after delivery.

THE ABDOMINAL MUSCLES

Structure of the abdominal muscles

The abdominal muscles are comprised of four layers: transversus abdominis, internal oblique, external oblique and rectus abdominis. These muscles are all interconnected to form a muscular corset.

Fig. 2.1	**Transversus abdominis**

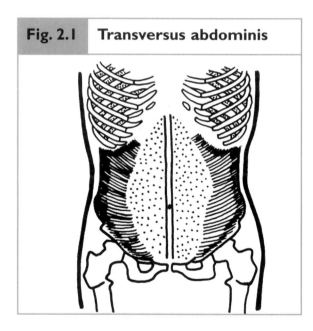

Transversus abdominis

Transversus abdominis (TrA) is the deepest of the four muscles. Starting in the thoracolumbar fascia of the back, the muscle wraps horizontally around the torso and the two sides insert into a broad tendinous band at the front called an aponeurosis. The aponeurosis of TrA joins with the aponeurosis of the obliques at the midline of the body to form the linea alba. As a result of this insertion TrA plays a significant role in stabilising the linea alba.

The linea alba is a tendinous raphe, seen along the midline of the abdomen between the inner borders of rectus abdominis. It is formed by the blending of the aponeurosis from both sides of the TrA and obliques. It is narrower below than above the umbilicus corresponding with the width of rectus abdominis as it descends.

Contraction of the TrA compresses and flattens the abdominal wall and draws the navel towards the spine. This action also pulls rectus abdominis towards the body and helps to reduce the separation of postnatal abdominals. Together with the obliques, TrA supports the internal organs and stabilizes the pelvis and lower spine. However, since TrA is frequently a very weak muscle it does not automatically contract alongside the other abdominals and must be consciously contracted to make it join in. This has important implications for all abdominal work.

Internal oblique

The internal oblique lies on top of the TrA muscle and forms an inverted V shape. Its origins are thoracolumbar fascia and iliac crest and its fibres run both inwards to the linea alba and upwards to the lower four ribs. As with TrA this muscle feeds into its own aponeurosis which forms part of the linea alba, as described above. The aponeurosis of the internal oblique is particularly significant as it subdivides at the outer edges of the rectus abdominis and passes

Fig. 2.2   Internal oblique

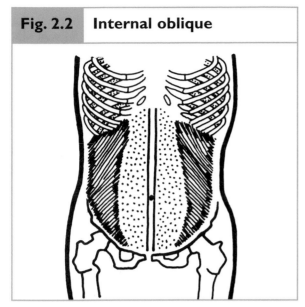

Fig. 2.3   External oblique

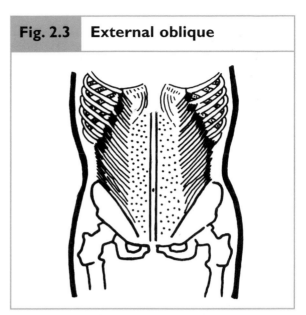

in front of and behind the rectus muscle, encasing it within a sheath, before re-joining at the linea alba. This occurs on the upper three-quarters of rectus abdominis only; in the lower quarter of the muscle the three layers of aponeurosis go over the top of rectus abdominis.

Due to the variable direction of its fibres, internal obliques can assist TrA with abdominal compression, flex the trunk to the same side and work with external obliques on the opposite side to provide trunk rotation.

External oblique

The external oblique lies on top of the internal oblique and forms an upright V shape. It originates on the lower eight ribs and runs diagonally and vertically downwards to insert onto the iliac crest. The midline attachment feeds into its own aponeurosis which passes over the top of rectus abdominis and meets with its opposite number in the centre to form the linea alba.

External obliques work together with internal obliques from the opposite side to

rotate the trunk. They also assist rectus abdominis with trunk flexion.

Rectus abdominis

The rectus abdominis (RA) forms the uppermost layer of the abdominal muscles. It is

Fig. 2.4   Rectus abdominis

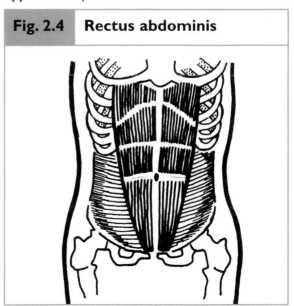

| **Fig. 2.5** | **Cross section of abdominal muscles** |

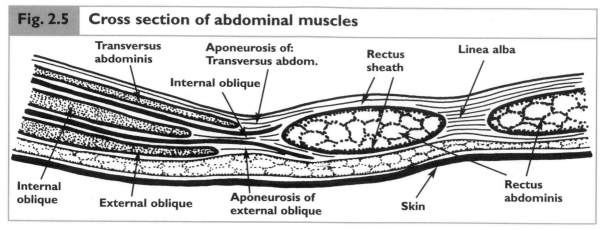

made up of two bands of muscle which begin on the pubic bone, and travel upwards to attach onto 5th, 6th, and 7th ribs. It is narrower at the bottom and increases in width to approximately 15 cm at the top. The muscle has three fibrous bands, known as tendinous inscriptions, that transverse it, one at the level of the umbilicus and two above it. This has particular relevance when checking for separation of the muscles (*see* page 27) as the area around the umbilicus is most vulnerable. Each side of RA is encased in a sheath made from the aponeurosis of the oblique and TrA muscles. These merge together in the centre to form the linea alba. In the lower quarter of the abdomen, the aponeurosis only covers the top of the recti muscles, which has implications for caesarean deliveries (*see* page 13).

Functions of the abdominal muscles

The abdominal muscles:

* stabilise and support the lumbar spine;
* support the abdominal and pelvic organs;
* flex the trunk to one side;
* curl the trunk upwards from a lying position;

* rotate the trunk;
* maintain correct pelvic alignment;
* brace the body under stress, e.g. lifting, coughing or sneezing;
* aid expulsive movements, e.g. vomiting, excretion and during the second stage of labour.

Pregnancy and the abdominal muscles

What happens to the abdominal muscles during pregnancy?

Under the influence of relaxin (*see* Chapter 1) the abdominal muscles undergo a tremendous amount of stretching in all directions. Connective tissue within the muscles themselves provides a degree of elasticity, but the main changes occur to the linea alba. The linea alba is connective tissue formed by the joining of the aponeurosis of the TrA and oblique muscles. Relaxin increases the water content of collagen fibres found within connective tissue, resulting in increased elasticity of the linea alba in both directions. The waistline may increase by approximately 50 cm (20 in) and rectus abdominis may lengthen by approximately 20 cm (8 in). The

Fig. 2.6	Abs during pregnancy

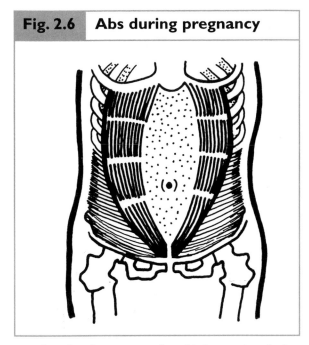

two bands of recti muscle which previously lay parallel stretch away from the midline to allow more space for the growing uterus (*see* Figure 2.6). This is known as diastasis recti – separation of the recti muscles – and is quite common, occurring in 66 per cent of women in the third trimester. Actual separation is not painful and many women will be unaware that it has happened, although they may have chronic backache due to lack of support from the abdominal muscles (*see* Chapter 5).

Stretch weakness

Stretch weakness occurs when a muscle remains elongated, beyond its normal resting position but within its normal range (Kendall et al. 1993). In this position, its contractile ability is reduced as the actin and myosin filaments are taken too far apart to contract. The muscle adapts by adding another sarcomere to the end of the muscle which pushes the contractile elements closer together.

This change occurs in rectus abdominis as it stretches over the pregnant uterus and results in weakness within the muscle's inner range (Norris 2000). Postnatally, muscle length will gradually reduce but can be speeded up by inner-range training (*see* page 26 for suitable exercises).

What happens to the abdominals during a caesarean section?

Trauma to the abdominal muscles during a caesarean section is not as severe as many women believe; the muscles themselves are not cut. An incision of approximately 10 cm is made just above the pubic bone which cuts through the rectus sheath and the two sides of the rectus muscle are drawn apart. As there is only one layer of aponeurosis in the lower portion of the abdomen, once the muscles have been separated sufficient space is created to proceed with the delivery. After the baby has been lifted out, the rectus sheath is repaired and the muscles realigned.

Is it more difficult for the muscles to recover after a caesarean?

Most women who deliver by caesarean section feel that abdominal recovery is inhibited by the procedure. Although the muscles themselves have not been cut, the layers of aponeurosis have; contraction of TrA may cause pain or discomfort that may inhibit effective engagement. Exercises for TrA should be encouraged as soon as possible and progressed slowly, provided no pain is felt. Trapped air, as a result of surgery, may add to the problem in the first couple of days post-delivery. This can be assisted by performing pelvic tilts in a supine position. Tingling and numbness will be experienced around the scar site, with sensation returning in patches; full sensory recovery could take up to six months.

How do the muscles repair after pregnancy?

Three to four days after the baby is born the recti muscles will begin to realign and the wide separation will gradually reduce. By six weeks the separation is usually about two finger widths apart or less (*see* notes on 'Rec check') but this will vary in some women, depending on how many pregnancies they have had and how strong the muscles were before pregnancy. Gentle exercises to encourage RA to shorten and come together will be invaluable in the early postnatal period and will speed up recovery time. These exercises – navel to spine contractions and pelvic tilting – are usually advised on discharge from hospital.

Care of the abdominal muscles

The abdominal muscles may remain stretched and weakened for some time after delivery, leaving the spine in a vulnerable position until full strength has been regained. Particular care should be taken to protect the abdominals and the back during everyday activities.

See Appendix.

Strengthening the abdominal muscles

How soon should abdominal exercises commence?

As soon as possible after delivery – ideally within 24 hours. Level 1A TrA and RA exercises (*see* pages ???) are suitable to do in the first few days after delivery and are generally those given out to women by the hospital on discharge. Drawing navel to spine should be practised as often as possible throughout the day. Four-point kneeling should be avoided

until after six weeks (*see* page 21).

What are the aims of postnatal abdominal recovery?

- To strengthen TrA to assist realignment of linea alba and increase core stability.
- To shorten RA and strengthen within its inner range.

Why are exercises for transversus abdominis so important?

TrA is a deep postural muscle. It is responsible for maintaining a strong, controlled centre to allow the limbs to move freely. Lack of stabilisation is a primary cause of lower back pain. Pregnancy reduces functional use of the abdominal wall resulting in postnatal vulnerability of the pelvis and lower back. Strong limbs held together by a weak centre cannot function effectively, and sooner or later injury will occur.

Postural recovery must begin with TrA

The essential first stage of abdominal recovery is to increase the strength of TrA. Navel to spine contractions should be practised in many different positions (i.e. side and supine lying, sitting or standing) so that these deep muscles can be strengthened to provide support for all functional movements. Re-education is crucial to the stability of all movements so it is important to dedicate sufficient time and emphasis to this muscle before progressing.

Locating transversus abdominis

- Standing or sitting place your fingers on your

hip bones at the front of the pelvis (ASIS) and move them diagonally downwards and inwards approx 2.5 cm.

- Apply gentle pressure into the soft tissue and cough several times.
- Feel the TrA muscle pushing outwards underneath your fingers as you cough.
- Repeat, but this time, perform a navel to spine contraction.
- Feel the difference these muscles make to the abdomen as they appear to thicken underneath towards your fingers and reduce movement of the abdominal wall during the cough.

Contracting transversus abdominis

Although it appears incredibly simple, this movement takes time to learn and perform correctly. Many women experience great difficulty in recruiting TrA without either holding their breath or co-contracting gluteus maximus and performing a posterior pelvic tilt. To effectively contract TrA and create sufficient stability for the spine, it only needs to contract 25 per cent of its maximum (Richardson et al 1995). A soft, sinking feeling, rather like a balloon deflating in the abdomen, is all that is required but many women will brace and pull strongly in whilst inhaling. This action recruits rectus abdominis and external obliques and overrides the action of TrA. Ribcage depression and a horizontal crease across the upper abdomen will indicate these muscles are being incorrectly used. Recent research suggests that TrA works most effectively in neutral spine (Sapsford et al. 2001) so adoption of this alignment is highly recommended where possible.

Transversus abdominis/pelvic floor link

In the past we have encouraged pelvic floor contractions to be performed in association with resisted abdominal work. This was felt necessary to avoid stressing the pelvic floor with increased abdominal pressure. Not only has this proved quite complex in practice but now appears to be unnecessary as research suggests that the pelvic floor muscles automatically contract with TrA (Sapsford et al. 2001). Activated by the same neural loop, it seems the TrA has reciprocal benefits when the pelvic floor is contracted. It is worth noting however, that if the abdominals are incorrectly braced when trying to achieve navel to spine, i.e. RA takes over the work, intra-abdominal pressure rises and forces the pelvic floor muscles downwards.

EXERCISES FOR TRANSVERSUS ABDOMINIS (Level 1A)

Standing exercises

Navel to spine contraction

Purpose: to shorten and strengthen the TrA muscles that stabilise the spine. This will help to flatten the abdomen and re-establish correct posture.

Preparation
In any position – sitting or standing.

Action
Inhale, and as you exhale draw navel gently

Ex 2.1	**Naval to spine contraction**

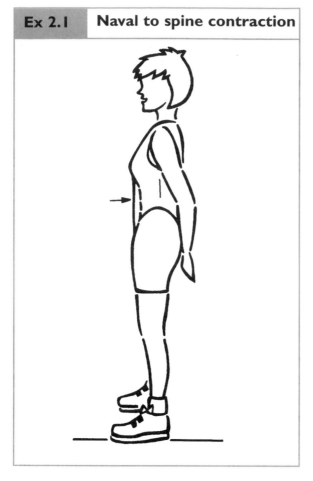

into spine. Hold for a few seconds and release without letting the abdomen push out. Repeat as often as possible throughout the day, gradually increasing the length of hold but continuing to breathe throughout.

Technique tips
- Make it a soft sinking feeling rather than a strong bracing action.
- Keep breathing throughout.
- As strength improves, increase the length of hold, progressing towards 20 seconds.
- Repeat this exercise as many times as possible throughout the day.

- Practise whilst feeding/changing baby, preparing food, walking with the pushchair, talking etc.
- Repetition will have a significant effect on abdominal recovery.

Floor exercises

Getting down to the floor
When bending down to sit or lie on the floor the following safety points should be considered.

- Neutral spine and draw in the abdominal muscles.
- Bend your knees rather than your back.

Side lying abdominal raise
Purpose: to strengthen the TrA muscles that stabilise the spine and assist with the maintenance of correct posture. This position is particularly helpful for muscle recruitment and is a good exercise to begin with.

Preparation
Side lying in a comfortable position with spine in neutral, knees together and bent to 45 degrees.

Action
Inhale to prepare, and as you exhale draw navel to spine and try to lift the abdomen away from the floor without moving the buttocks or the back. Inhale to release with control.

Technique tips
- Avoid tilting the pelvis to create the movement.
- Feel the abdomen lifting upwards and inwards.

- Keep the upper body relaxed.
- Keep the breath natural.

Progression
Hold the contraction whilst continuing to breathe. Release when control wavers.

Front lying abdominal raise

Purpose: to strengthen the TrA muscles that stabilise the spine and assist with the maintenance of correct posture.

Preparation
Lie prone (if you are comfortable) with your hands under forehead, head in line with body. Relax the abdomen into the floor.

Action
Keeping the rest of the body relaxed, inhale, and as you exhale draw navel to spine and try to lift the abdomen off the floor. Avoid squeezing the buttocks or pelvic tilting. Aim to hold for a count of six, continuing to breathe. Release with control, letting the abdomen relax into the floor.

Technique tips
- Keep your pubic and hips bones in contact with the floor.
- Feel your abdomen gently lifting away from the floor.

- Breathe throughout.
- Tilting the pelvis will involve the rectus abdominis muscle and will not work the transversus muscle in isolation as intended.
- If your breasts feel uncomfortable try performing this exercise in a kneeling position. **NB** See page 21 'Caution'.

Caution: Do not press down with the arms to take the pressure off the breasts as this may cause the back to overextend.

Moving to supine lying

Always roll on to your side before gently moving on to your back. Keep your knees and feet together with abdominal muscles lightly drawn in, and turn the whole body as one. Rolling the legs before the upper body will twist the lower back and pull on the oblique muscles.

Finding supine neutral spinal alignment

Before commencing any supine exercises it is essential to align the spine correctly.

- Lie on your back with knees bent and feet flat on the floor, hip-width apart.
  NB Hip width should be taken from the position of ASIS (hip bones) and not the outside of the thighs.

Ex 2.2	Front lying abdominal raise

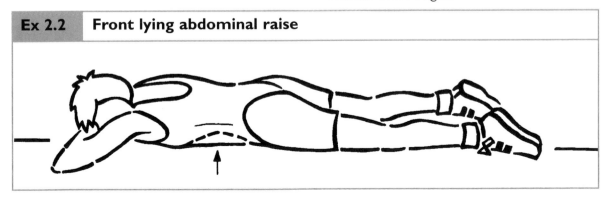

Ex 2.3	Neutral spinal alignment

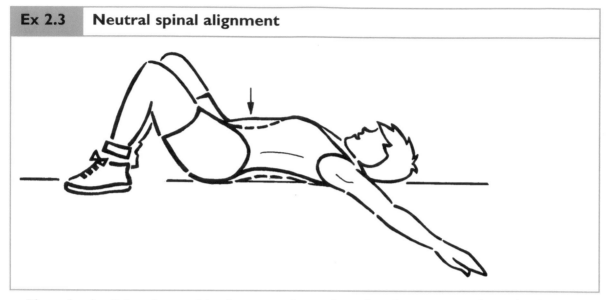

- Place heel of hands on hip bones and fingertips on pubic bone.
- Gently roll the pelvis forward (pubic bone downwards) so that your back arches off the floor and fingertips lower.
- Gently roll the pelvis the opposite way so that your lower back presses into the floor and the fingertips lift.
- Find a position midway between these two extremes where the lower back forms a natural curve and heel of hands/fingertips are on the same horizontal plane.
- This is your neutral spine position.

Note: adopting the neutral spine position only involves movement of the bones. There should be no muscular contraction involved in holding you there. Allow yourself a few seconds to relax into this position. Then go through the following checkpoints:

- Equal weight between right and left foot
- Buttocks, front of thighs and lower back relaxed
- Shoulder-blades sliding down your back
- Arms lengthening away from shoulders
- Breastbone relaxed
- Nose in line with breastbone and pubic bone
- Spine long

Leg slides

Purpose: to use the TrA to stabilise the pelvis whilst moving the legs.

Preparation
Lie supine with neutral spinal alignment as before.

Ex 2.4	Leg slide

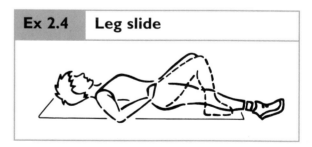

Action
Inhale to prepare and as you exhale draw navel to spine and slide one leg out along the floor

until the knee straightens. Inhale to hold, exhale to draw navel to spine and slide the leg back up to the starting position.

Technique tips
- Lengthen the leg away from the hip.
- Avoid rocking the pelvis.
- Keep the ribcage down into the floor.
- Keep the upper body stable throughout.

Scissor arms

Purpose: to mobilise the shoulder girdle and ribcage, using TrA to stabilise the torso. This exercise also assists the lower ribs return to their pre-pregnancy position, which is important for waistline remodelling.

Preparation
Lie supine with neutral spinal alignment as before.

Ex 2.5	Scissor arms

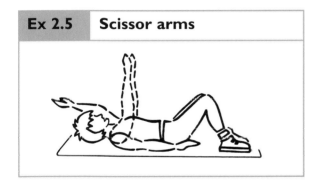

Action
Inhale and float both arms up towards the ceiling at chest height, keeping the shoulder blades into the floor. Exhale, drawing navel to spine, and lengthen the right arm above the head and left arm down by your side. Keep the ribcage down into the floor. Inhale to return both arms to ceiling at chest height. Breathe out and repeat, changing arms.

Technique tips
- Maintain neutral spine throughout by gently drawing in the abdominal muscles.
- Range of movement of the arm is determined by the ability to keep the ribcage on the floor. This may be only a small movement for some people – if the ribcage begins to lift the arm has gone too far and stabilisation is lost.
- Think of moving the arms from the centre of the back, rather than the shoulders themselves.
- Get a feeling of lengthening the arms away from the shoulders.

Progression
Combine this exercise with leg slide, using opposite arm and leg.

Chest flye

Purpose: to mobilise the shoulder girdle and ribcage, using TrA to stabilise the torso. This exercise is also helpful for rib closure.

Preparation
Supine, neutral spinal alignment as before.

Ex 2.6	Chest flye

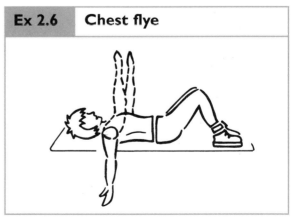

Action
Inhale and lift both arms towards the ceiling at

chest height. Release the shoulders and allow the shoulder blades to sink into the floor. Exhale, drawing navel softly to spine, as you open both arms out to the side towards the floor, keeping the ribcage and shoulder blades drawing down. Inhale to return both arms up towards the ceiling.

Technique tips
- Be sure to engage TrA as the arms open to the side, this will maintain neutral spinal alignment – avoid squeezing the buttocks.
- Keep the ribs in contact with the floor.
- Think of moving from the centre of the back rather than the shoulders.
- Lengthen the arms out and away from the shoulders.

Arm circles

Purpose: to mobilise the shoulder girdle and ribcage, using TrA to stabilise the torso. This exercise is also helpful for rib closure.

Preparation
Supine, neutral spinal alignment as before.

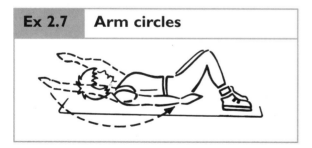

Ex 2.7 **Arm circles**

Action
Inhale and lift both arms towards the ceiling at chest height. Release the shoulders and allow the shoulder blades to sink into the floor. Exhale, drawing navel softly to spine, and float the arms overhead, keeping the ribcage into the floor. Inhale as you circle both arms around to

the side and down, drawing shoulders blades down, and continue the movement until the arms are above chest. Repeat.

Technique tips
- Get a feeling of scooping the air as the arms press gently around.
- Keep shoulder blades drawing down throughout.
- Do not allow the ribcage to lift as the arms go above the head.

Progression (Level 2)
Combine with leg glide.

Bent knee fall-out

Purpose: to challenge TrA to maintain neutral spine.

Preparation
Lie supine, in neutral spinal alignment. Elbows bent with fingertips resting on hip bones.

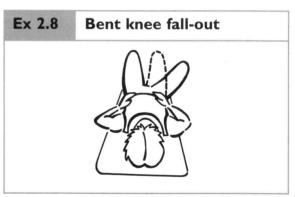

Ex 2.8 **Bent knee fall-out**

Action
Inhale, and as you exhale draw navel to spine and open the right knee to the side without moving the pelvis. Inhale to hold, exhale to draw navel to spine and return the knee up to starting position. Repeat on the other side.

Technique tips
- Keep the pelvis level throughout – check this with hands on hips.
- Take the leg only as far as you can maintain correct pelvic alignment.
- Do not allow the other knee to drop out to counterbalance the movement – keep it pointing up to the ceiling.
- Draw the ribcage down into the floor as the leg moves away to maintain spinal alignment.
- Keep the upper body relaxed throughout.
- Lengthen your arms away from the shoulders.
- Perform slowly and with control.

Caution: Stop immediately any discomfort is felt in the symphysis pubis or sacroiliac joints.

Knee raise

Purpose: to use TrA to stabilise the torso whilst lifting the knees.

Preparation
Lie supine in neutral spinal alignment as before.

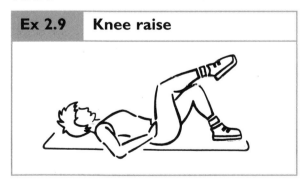

Ex 2.9	Knee raise

Action
Inhale to prepare, and as you exhale draw navel to spine and lift one foot off the floor, bringing your knee up over the hip. Inhale to hold, exhale to keep navel to spine as you lower

the foot to the floor, keeping your spine in the same position. TrA is working hard to maintain neutral alignment of the spine as you lift and lower the leg.

Technique tips
- Maintain neutral alignment throughout.
- Use the abdominals to prevent the pelvis rocking as the foot lifts.
- Avoid pressing down onto the supporting foot.
- Keep the upper body relaxed.
- Keep shoulder-blades sliding down.

EXERCISES FOR TRANSVERSUS ABDOMINIS (Level 1B TrA)

Kneeling exercises

Caution: The Association of Chartered Physiotherapists in Women's Health recommend that exercises in the four-point kneeling position should be postponed until six weeks after delivery. There is a small risk of air entering the circulation through the raw placental site, before this time, causing an embolus.

Finding neutral spinal alignment in four-point kneeling

This position is frequently incorrectly adopted as it is quite difficult for individuals to find for themselves – instructor observation is essential. Moving through anterior and posterior pelvic tilts should be performed in a slow, controlled way.

- Knees under hips and hands under shoulders, fingers facing forward.

- Roll the pelvis downwards so the tailbone lifts and lumbar lordosis increases.
- Roll the pelvis the opposite way so the back curls towards the ceiling.
- Find a position midway between these two extremes where the lower back forms a natural curve.
- Push gently away from the hands without flexing thoracic spine.
- Slide the shoulder-blades down.
- Lift head to be in line with sacrum and mid-thoracic spine.
- Distribute weight equally between knees and hands.
- Buttocks, front of thighs and lower back relaxed.
- Spine long.
- Draw navel to spine.

Kneeling abdominal raise

Purpose: as for the front lying abdominal raise.

Preparation
On hands and knees, in neutral alignment as described above.

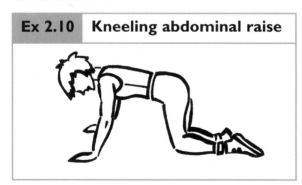

| Ex 2.10 | Kneeling abdominal raise |

Action
Inhale, and as you exhale draw navel to spine to gently lift the abdomen. Keep the elbows slightly bent to prevent them locking. Hold for a count of six, continuing to breathe. Lower with control to the starting position, taking care

not to let the back arch.

Technique tips
- Tilting the pelvis will involve RA and will not work TrA in isolation as intended.
- If you find this position uncomfortable due to tingling or numbness in the fingers you could try resting your elbows on a chair in a kneeling position, or perform the front lying version described on page 17 if this is more comfortable.

Kneeling leg and arm raise

Purpose: to use TrA to stabilise the torso whilst moving the arms or legs.

Preparation
On hands and knees, in neutral alignment as described above.

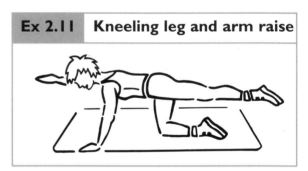

| Ex 2.11 | Kneeling leg and arm raise |

Action
Perform the following as two separate movements:

1 Inhale to prepare. As you exhale, draw navel to spine and slide one foot out along the floor, lengthening the leg away from you. Do not allow the pelvis to tip. Inhale to hold, as you exhale draw navel to spine and slide the leg slowly back in again. Repeat both sides.
2 Repeat the navel to spine sequence and slide the arm forward, lengthening from the

fingertips as the arms lifts. Aim to lift it parallel to the floor, sliding the shoulder-blades down and maintaining neutral spine.

Progression (Level 2)
- Combine the two movements using opposite arm and leg.
- As above, but lift the leg off the floor.

EXERCISES FOR TRANSVERSUS ABDOMINIS (Level 2A)

Table top exercises

Some exercises in this section are performed from 'table top' position. True table top involves positioning the knees above the hips with spine in neutral. However, to ensure spinal safety at this stage, it is essential to use the modified version where knees remain over chest and lower back is in contact with the floor. This allows a safe margin of error so that participants will move into neutral rather than hyperextension if correct alignment cannot be maintained. Once strength has been gained, these exercises can all be progressed to a neutral table top – some are extremely demanding to perform correctly in this position. Progress must be slow.

Ex 2.12	Table top

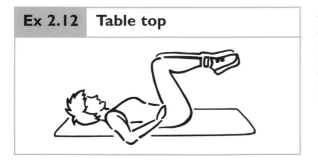

Moving into table top position
- Inhale to prepare, and as you exhale draw navel to spine and lift one foot off the floor, bringing knee up over chest.
- Allow the pelvis to tilt so the lower back makes contact with the floor.
- Repeat, lifting the other knee up to join, maintaining back alignment.
- Draw knees together and ensure the lower legs are parallel to the floor.

NB To prevent hyperextension on the transition, it may be necessary to use the hands to hold the first knee in position before lifting the second knee.

Toe touch

Purpose: to challenge TrA to stabilise the torso whilst lifting and lowering the legs.

Preparation
In table top position as above, arms relaxed by sides.

Ex 2.13	Toe touch

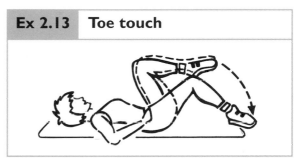

Action
As you exhale draw navel to spine and lower the right foot to the floor, keeping the back into the floor. Inhale to rest on the floor, exhale to keep navel to spine and lift the leg back up. Change legs and repeat on the other side.

Technique tips
- With both legs lifted the TrA has to work harder to maintain spinal alignment.
- Press the ribcage down into the floor as the leg lowers to maintain alignment.
- Do not allow the pelvis to roll forward as the leg lowers.
- Keep the abdomen flat.
- Keep the upper body relaxed throughout.
- Lengthen your arms away from the shoulders.

NB If discomfort is felt in the lower back, use your arms to hold the stationary knee towards your chest. This will assist the abdominals to keep the back in correct alignment.

Progression
- Touch the tips of the toes lightly on the floor rather than resting the foot down.
- When TrA strength increases this exercise should be performed from neutral, i.e. knees over hips, and neutral spinal alignment maintained for the duration of the sequence.

Leg glide

Purpose: to challenge TrA to maintain spinal alignment.

Preparation
In table top position as above, arms relaxed by sides.

Action
Inhale to prepare, and as you exhale draw navel to spine and slowly glide your knees away from your chest, towards the vertical, keeping the back into the floor. Inhale to draw the legs back to start position. The further the legs are taken away from the chest the harder the abdominals have to work to prevent the back arching off the floor.

Technique tips
- Draw the ribcage down into the floor as the legs move away to maintain spinal alignment.
- Do not allow the pelvis to roll forward with the legs.
- Keep the abdomen flat.
- Keep the lower legs parallel to floor.
- Keep the upper body relaxed throughout.
- Lengthen your arms away from the shoulders.
- This exercise can also be performed with feet resting on a stability ball.

Progression
When strength increases, this exercise can be performed from neutral. The movement should be very small, 3–6 cm with spinal alignment maintained.

Caution: Stop immediately and review technique if discomfort is felt in the lower back.

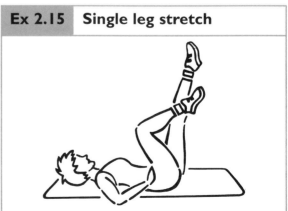

Ex 2.15 | **Single leg stretch**

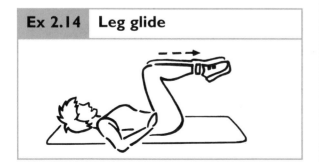

Ex 2.14 | **Leg glide**

Single leg stretch

Purpose: to challenge TrA to maintain spinal alignment.

Preparation
In table top position as above, arms relaxed by sides.

Action
Inhale, and as you exhale draw navel to spine and extend one leg towards the ceiling, drawing the other knee further into the chest. Exhale to change legs, moving both legs simultaneously and keeping the back into the floor. Keep the top leg slightly bent to avoid pulling on the hamstrings. Once co-ordination has been achieved, the top leg can be lowered from vertical, a little way towards the floor (approx. 60 degrees)

Technique tips
- The outward pull of the leg challenges the abdominals to keep the back in the same position on the floor.
- Focus on breathing out and drawing navel to spine with each extension – the inhalation will occur naturally.
- Keep the abdomen flat.
- Draw the ribcage down into the floor as the legs move away to maintain spinal alignment.
- Do not allow the pelvis to roll forward with the leg.
- Avoid locking knees.
- Keep the upper body relaxed throughout.
- Lengthen the arms away from the shoulders.

Caution: If discomfort is felt in the lower back keep the top leg lifted higher. Taking the leg too low will cause the lower back to buckle from the floor if the abdominals are not strong enough to support.

Knee roll

Purpose: to challenge TrA to maintain neutral spine.

Caution: This exercise is unsuitable for women with sacroiliac problems or those with an RA separation wider than two fingers.

Preparation
Lie supine in neutral spinal alignment with knees bent up, feet flat on the floor.

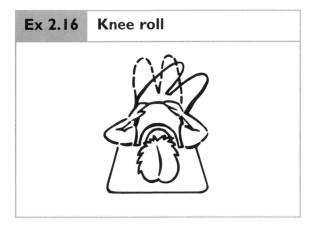

Ex 2.16   Knee roll

Action
Inhale to prepare, and as you exhale draw navel to spine and allow the knees to roll over to one side, towards the floor. Keep the feet and buttocks firmly on the floor. Inhale to hold and as you exhale keep navel to spine and use the abdominals to draw your knees back into position.

Technique tips
- Maintain neutral alignment throughout.
- Keep both buttocks firmly into the floor.
- Draw the ribcage from the opposite side down into the floor to help recover.
- Only go as far as the legs remain controlled.
- Keep the abdomen flat.

EXERCISE FOR TRANSVERSUS ABDOMINIS (Level 2B)

NB Not to be performed before six weeks (*see* page 21).

Modified plank

Purpose: to challenge TrA to stabilise the torso.

Preparation
Lie prone with upper body lifted onto forearms, elbows bent under shoulders and palms facing inwards.

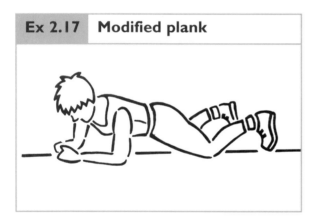

Ex 2.17 | **Modified plank**

Action
Inhale to prepare and as you exhale draw navel to spine and lift the abdomen off the floor, maintaining neutral spine. Hold for a few seconds, continuing to breathe. Lower with control.

Technique tips
• Maintain navel to spine throughout.
• Draw shoulder-blades down and lengthen the spine.

• Keep the head aligned with the spine.
• Keep the hip bones on the floor.

Progression
• Repeat, lifting the hip bones off the floor.
• Bend the knees in towards the buttocks and repeat, lifting the pubic bone off the floor – this is a Level 3 exercise.

Why do you need to shorten rectus abdominis?

The overstretched RA muscle must be shortened before strengthening can begin. If strengthening exercises commence before the muscles have realigned or before TrA has been strengthened, then doming will occur during a curl-up (see below).

Which exercises will help to shorten rectus abdominis?

• Posterior pelvic tilting in as many positions as possible will draw the two ends of the muscle closer together.
• Working RA within its 'inner range', i.e. Half roll back or curl up and hold.

Perform the 'rec check' before commencing rectus abdominis work

It is important to check the condition of RA to determine how far apart the two sides of the muscle are lying. Commencing resisted RA work with a wide separation will impair abdominal recovery. Results will depend on several factors: abdominal condition prior to pregnancy, the process of labour and delivery, and the amount and type of exercise performed since delivery – TrA work, it is hoped.

How to test for separation of rectus abdominis

The 'rec check'

Preparation

Lie on your back with your knees bent up and feet flat on the floor. Adjust your positioning so that the spine is in correct neutral alignment (*see* page 17). Relax the abdomen and place two fingers of one hand sideways across the abdomen around the area of the umbilicus. Apply gentle pressure to the abdomen.

Action

Inhale to prepare, and as you exhale draw navel to spine and slowly raise head and shoulders off the floor, keeping gentle pressure on the abdomen with the fingertips. Hold, continuing to breathe, and register the sensation felt under the fingertips. Lower with control keeping navel to spine.

Explanation

- As the head and shoulders lift you should be able to feel the two bands of recti muscle closing in around the fingers. They will feel like hard ridges on either side of the fingers with the soft dip* of the linea alba in the centre.
- If this cannot be felt, it may be necessary to curl up a little higher.
- If the gap between the two muscle bands appears to be wider than two fingers, repeat the test using three fingers.
- Repeat the test just below the umbilicus – the reading may be different.
- Check several times until you are sure of the result.

* Connective tissue between the two bands of recti muscle will still be stretched and weak so the fingers will sink deeply into the abdomen during this test.

Teaching the 'rec check'

When teaching this to a client, it is essential to explain clearly the purpose of the test and how the results will affect her recovery, as a hands-on experience like this may not be welcomed by some women.

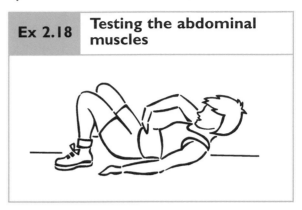

Ex 2.18 **Testing the abdominal muscles**

It is helpful to explain the location of RA and the changes it has undergone during pregnancy. The explanation can be complemented by demonstrating with a zip (approx. 50 cm long) showing the points of attachment on to the pubis and sternum, and how the two sides of the muscle stretch away from the midline as pregnancy increases. The zip can also be used to clarify how the shortening of these muscles encourages them back into correct alignment. This visual aid improves understanding of a rather complex concept. It is vital that individuals understand exactly what they are feeling for so that when the hard ridges of muscle butt against the side of the fingers they can distinguish between this and the soft, pliable centre. Re-testing at a later date is excellent confirmation of progress. Some women may dislike pushing their fingers into their abdomen, particularly around the umbilicus, and may feel very sensitive about performing the test. Most women will want clarification of their findings, particularly those with minimal separation, as it will be more difficult to palpate. An instructor should always wait to be asked by the individual and avoid performing the check without gaining permission first.

How wide should the separation be?

By six weeks the separation may be the width of two fingers or less. If the gap is wider than this, the muscles can still recover providing the correct exercises are performed (see TrA exercises). Even when fully recovered the muscles will always lie slightly apart (approximately 1.5–2 cm).

Which exercises can be performed if the separation is wider than two fingers?

- Navel to spine in as many positions as possible. **NB** Avoid four-point kneeling until after six weeks.
- Pelvic tilting in as many positions as possible (except four-point kneeling prior to six weeks).
- Level 1A TrA exercises.
- Gentle head and shoulder raising to the point before 'doming' occurs (see below). Ensure the abdominal muscles remain pulled in throughout to reduce the chances of doming occurring.

Should any exercises be avoided?

Exercises for the oblique muscles must be avoided due to their insertion into the aponeurosis. Any exercise or activity that involves strong rotation or side flexion should also be avoided for the same reason. Additionally, movements that stretch the abdominals are inappropriate; the emphasis must be on shortening the overstretched muscles. Exercises in the four-point kneeling position should be avoided until after six weeks.

Doming

Doming is a bulge in the abdominal wall that occurs when there is still separation of RA. If the TrA muscle is not strong enough to maintain abdominal compression as RA contracts, internal pressure pushes the underneath tissue up between the two recti muscles creating a doming effect on the abdomen.

Is doming harmful to the abdominal muscles?

If doming continues during a curl-up, the two bands of recti muscle may not realign in parallel and this may jeopardise abdominal recovery. It is more likely to occur around the umbilicus as it is the joining site of the linea alba vertically and the lower tendinous band horizontally – the weakest point.

Which exercises can be performed if the separation is less than two fingers?

TrA will be weak in every woman, even with a small separation. *Always* begin with the Level 1A exercises for both TrA and RA – full recovery will be hampered if this vital stage is omitted. Whilst low-level resisted RA exercises can be commenced (most women are desperate to start these as soon as possible) it should be explained that these will not flatten the abdomen. A combination of both will successfully meet the aims of abdominal recovery explained earlier.

Can twisting curls for the oblique muscles be introduced now?

Due to their structure it is advisable to concentrate on restoring strength to the other abdominal muscles before commencing work on the obliques. It is important to stabilise the linea alba by shortening and strengthening the TrA and then to gain strength in the RA with head and shoulder raises, progressing to knee reaches as in basic curls. Only then, when strength and stability has returned, should work on the obliques be introduced.

Why is correct breathing so important for abdominal work?

Correct breathing can enhance muscular focus by encouraging a low effort TrA response.

Regular practice of navel to spine contractions on exhalation will encourage the TrA to engage automatically. As a result, the pelvic floor, diaphragm and multifidus (via its attachment into the thoracolumbar fascia), are co-activated, increasing intra-abdominal pressure and providing additional support to the spine.

Incorrect head position

Soreness and discomfort in the neck is frequently experienced with abdominal work to the degree that the neck often tires before the abdominals. This is due to overflexing the neck (chin tucked tightly into chest) or extending the neck (pushing the chin forward) to try and assist the movement. The role of the neck muscles in a curl-up is to stabilise the head in its correct alignment while RA provides flexion of the spine. Neck discomfort may be compounded by tension already experienced in the upper body from feeding.

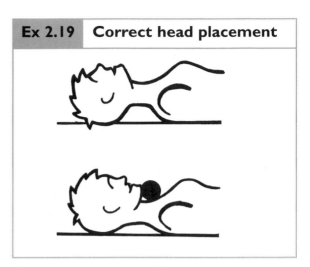

Ex 2.19 Correct head placement

Correct head position

Keeping the head relaxed on the floor, lengthen through the back of the neck so that the chin draws down towards the chest but is not tucked tightly inwards. Relax the shoulders and slide them down your back keeping the length through the back of the neck as you curl the ribs towards the hips. An excellent aid is to hold the baby's squeaky toy under the chin without squeaking or dropping it. Additionally, by placing the tongue on the roof of the mouth.

Alternatively, perform reduced repetitions of head and shoulder raises followed by pelvic tilting to rest the neck. If soreness continues, one hand can be placed behind the head for support but care must be taken to avoid pulling the head forward into incorrect alignment as the body curls. This hand position increases the intensity of the exercise and the abdominal muscles may tire sooner. A modified version of the reverse curl could also be performed as this exercise does not involve raising the head and shoulders off the floor. Correct, controlled technique is essential.

EXERCISES FOR RECTUS ABDOMINIS (Level 1A)

Floor exercises

Supine pelvic tilt

Purpose: to shorten rectus abdominis.

Preparation

Lie on your back with knees bent, feet flat on the floor in line with hip bones, and spine in neutral alignment (*see* page 17 for full alignment points).

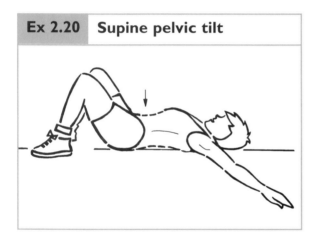

Ex 2.20	Supine pelvic tilt

Action

Inhale, and as you exhale draw navel to spine and tilt the pelvis so the pubic bone lifts. Feel your back pressing lightly into the floor. Hold, continuing to breathe. Release with control to the neutral spine position.

Technique tips

- Feel the abdomen scooping in towards the spine.
- Avoid squeezing the buttocks – try to make the abdominals do the work.

- Relax the shoulders and upper body as you exhale.
- Focus the work between the pubic bone and waist.
- Do not allow the back to over-arch on release.

Bridge

Purpose: to use RA to articulate the spine, and gluteus maximus and hamstrings to assist. This is also an excellent exercise for increasing spinal movements and mobilising stiff backs.

Preparation

Lying supine, with neutral spinal alignment, arms resting by your sides.

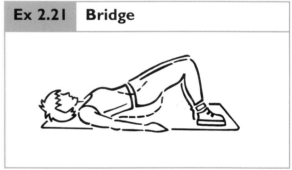

Ex 2.21	Bridge

Action

Pelvic tilt as above, then deepen the abdominal work so the spine begins to peel off the floor one vertebra at a time, exhaling as you lift. Feel the ribcage pressing down into the floor and pause when the tips of the shoulder-blades are just off the floor. Keeping the buttocks lifted, inhale, and as you exhale draw navel to spine, hinge at the ribcage and lower, slowly down to the floor, one vertebra at a time. Release and return to neutral spine.

Technique tips

- Use the abdominals to create the movement.

- Try to separate each vertebra and make individual contact with the floor.
- Pause in the lifted position forming a diagonal line between knees and shoulders.
- Draw the ribcage down.
- Do not lift onto the neck.
- Scoop the abdominal muscles to aid spinal flexion.
- Slow down through any tight areas to increase the range of movement.
- Lengthen the tailbone away from the head as you lower.
- Draw shoulder-blades down into the floor as you lower to avoid hunching the upper body.

Caution: Avoid over-squeezing the buttocks and gripping in the hamstrings as this may induce cramp.

Progressions of this exercise to challenge gluteus maximus are shown on page 106.

EXERCISES FOR RECTUS ABDOMINIS (Level IB)

Caution: Not to be performed before six weeks.

Kneeling pelvic tilt

Purpose: to shorten RA.

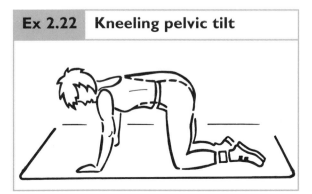

Ex 2.22	Kneeling pelvic tilt

Preparation
In four-point kneeling (*see* page 21) with neutral alignment.

Action
Inhale, and as you exhale draw navel to spine and pelvic tilt, curling the tail bone under, to bring hips closer to ribs. Keep the elbows slightly bent to prevent them locking. Hold for a few seconds, continuing to breathe. Lower with control to the starting position, taking care not to let the back arch.

Technique tips
- Use rectus abdominis to create the movement, avoid squeezing the buttocks.
- Focus the work from the pubic bone to the waist – avoid rounding in the upper back.
- Lengthen tailbone away from head as it curls under.
- Keep the shoulder-blades sliding down.
- If you find this position uncomfortable due to tingling or numbness in the fingers you could try resting your elbows on a chair in a kneeling position.

Adaptation
Take the movement further by rounding the back towards the ceiling, drawing ribs closer to hips and curling the head downwards. This is a lovely stretch for the spine.

EXERCISES FOR RECTUS ABDOMINIS (Level 2)

The following exercises gradually increase in intensity. Do not move on to the next stage until you have achieved and maintained the recommended level. Progression should be slow and gradual.

Stage I

Head and shoulder raise

Purpose: to strengthen RA and use TrA to stabilise the spine.

Preparation
Lie supine in neutral spinal alignment, hands on the floor beside you.

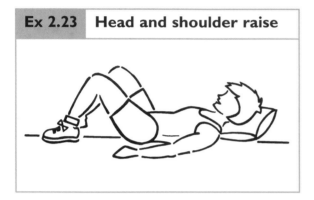

Ex 2.23	Head and shoulder raise

Action
Inhale and lengthen the back of the head along the floor, drawing the head into correct alignment (*see* page 29). As you exhale, draw navel to spine, and curl your ribcage towards your hips, raising head and shoulders off the floor. Keep the head in line with the spine as you lift. Inhale to hold, keeping the abdomen flat. Exhale, keeping navel to spine and lower with control to neutral starting position.

Technique tips
- Think of creating the movement from the ribcage rather than the head and shoulders.
- Reach the arms towards the feet as you curl.
- Keep the neck long and the shoulders-blades down.
- Keep the abdomen flat throughout.
- Do not allow the abdomen to dome.
- Avoid gripping in the hips.

- You may find it more comfortable to place a cushion underneath your head initially – move it away when you begin to feel stronger.

Caution: Curl up only to the point where the abdomen can be held in flat; if doming occurs the curl must be kept lower.

Head and shoulder raise with pelvic tilt

Purpose: to shorten and strengthen RA and use TrA to stabilise the spine.
NB This exercise encourages RA to shorten. Once this has occurred, head and shoulder raises should be performed from neutral.

Preparation
Lie supine with pelvis tilted, so the lower back presses gently into the floor, hands on the floor beside you.

Action
As above, maintaining the pelvic tilt throughout the repetitions. This exercise can be progressed by pelvic tilting with each lift and releasing to neutral alignment each time. Care should be taken that this does not allow the back to overextend on release.

Half roll back

Purpose: to strengthen RA within its inner range to aid muscle shortening and to challenge TrA to maintain abdominal compression. This exercise is often preferable to curl-ups due to reduced stress in the neck and shoulders.

Preparation
Sitting up on sit bones with knees bent, feet flat on the floor and spine in neutral alignment. Place hands under thighs but do not grip.

Ex 2.24	Half roll back

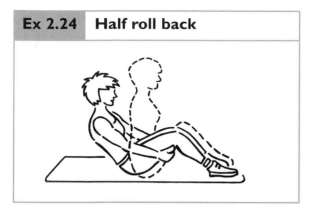

Action

Inhale to prepare and as you exhale draw navel to spine and tilt the pelvis, scooping the abdominals and lifting the pubic bone up as you roll off your sit bones onto the upper part of the buttocks. Avoid pulling on the thighs with your hands. Pause, continuing to breathe and maintain navel to spine. Return to upright sitting. Gradually increase the length of hold to 30 seconds.

Technique tips
- Create a C shape through the back.
- Avoid collapsing into the lower back – think of lengthening whilst curling.
- Release the shoulders and keep the head aligned.
- Maintain navel to spine connection.
- Use the abdominals to create the pelvic tilt.
- It may be necessary to squeeze the buttocks to achieve correct position.
- Keep the abdomen flat.
- Return to seated if the abdominals start to quiver.

Caution: If the abdomen begins to dome, return to the starting position and try again, ensuring navel has been drawn to spine. If doming continues reduce the range of movement. If discomfort is felt in the lower back reduce the range of movement.

Progression
- Take away the hand support and extend your arms out in front at chest height. Range of movement may need to be reduced to maintain technique.
- Once this can be comfortably achieved increase the range of movement by curling back a little further.
- Hold in the rolled-back position and perform a few repetitions of the scissor arms exercise (*see* page 19).

Stage II

Reverse curls

Purpose: to strengthen RA and use TrA to stabilise the spine. This exercise is particularly appropriate if discomfort is experienced in the neck during the previous abdominal exercises.

Preparation
Lie supine with knees lifted to tabletop position, (*see* p. 23) hands on the floor by your sides, palms down.

Ex 2.25	Reverse curls

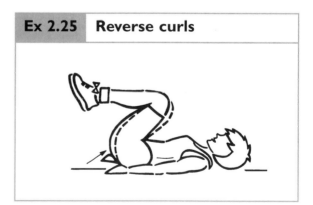

Action
Inhale to prepare, and as you exhale draw navel to spine and roll your hips towards your ribs with a slow squeezing action. Press gently

down with your hands to assist the movement. Inhale to roll gently down again keeping the knees bent in towards the chest.

Technique tips
- Keep knees into chest, as still as possible – swinging the legs will reduce the amount of work on the abdominals and make the movement uncontrolled.
- Maintain navel to spine connection.
- Scoop the abdominals in further to increase the movement.
- Roll pubic bone towards chest and try to lift your tailbone off the floor.
- Make it a slow squeezing action rather than a sudden hitch.
- Keep the knees over the chest as you lower.

Caution: This is an intensive exercise for the abdominals and should be performed only with the assistance of the arms during the early weeks. Knees must remain over the chest at all times to avoid hyperextension on release.

Progressions – Stage III
- Turn palms to ceiling to reduce the assistance of the arms.
- Slow down the movement.
- Cross arms over chest.

Stage III

Curl-up with hold

Purpose: to strengthen RA within its inner range and use TrA to stabilise the spine.

Preparation
Lying supine, with neutral spinal alignment, arms resting by your sides.

Action
Inhale to lengthen the back of the neck, and as you exhale draw navel to spine and slide ribs towards hips as you curl. Hold for a few seconds in the lifted position, continuing to breathe and maintaining navel to spine connection. Lower slowly to the starting position, keeping the abdomen flat.

Technique tips
- As for head and shoulder raise.
- Try to maintain the height of the curl during the hold.
- Feel the abdomen pulling in further during the hold.
- Support the head with one hand if strain is felt in the neck during the hold.
- Breathe throughout, particularly during the hold.
- If the position cannot be held, focus on a very slow lowering.

Caution: Stop immediately if the abdomen begins to bulge outwards during the hold and keep the curl lower for future repetitions.

Progression – Stage IV
Instructor assists into a higher lifted position which must then be held, unassisted, for as long as possible (building slowly to 30 seconds), and lower with control. Abdomen must be held flat.

EXERCISES FOR RECTUS ABDOMINIS Level 3

One hand to head

Purpose: to strengthen RA and use TrA to stabilise the spine.

Preparation
Lying supine, with neutral spinal alignment. One hand placed behind the head, other arm lengthened towards feet.

Ex 2.26 One hand to head

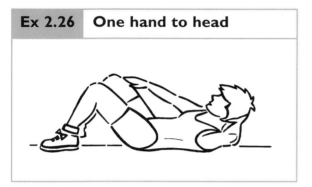

Action
As for head and shoulder raise, with one hand remaining behind the head, elbow facing outwards. Change arms after a few repetitions.

Technique tips
- As before.
- Relax the head into the hands.
- Maintain neutral spine.
- Keep the abdomen flat.

Caution: Do not pull the head forwards as you lift (*see* correct head placement page 29).

Progressions
- When this exercise begins to feel easier, you can increase the intensity again by placing both hands behind the head.
- The slower the exercise is performed the more difficult it is.

Twisting curl-up

Purpose: to strengthen internal and external oblique muscles and use TrA to stabilise the spine.

Caution: This exercise should be performed only if the abdomen can be held flat when performing the previous abdominal exercises. If the muscles dome this exercise must be avoided.

Preparation
Lying supine, with neutral spinal alignment. Right arm out straight to the side at shoulder height and the left hand on right thigh.

Ex 2.27 Twisting curl up

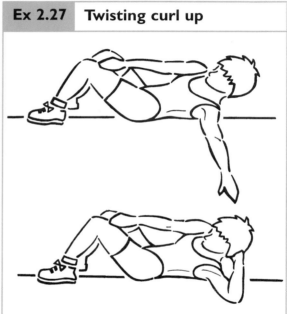

Action
Inhale to lengthen the back of the neck, and as you exhale draw navel to spine and curl left ribs towards right hip reaching the left hand to the outside of the right thigh (aim for the knee). Inhale to lower with control, keeping the abdomen held in. Repeat several times before changing to the other side.

Technique tips
- Keep both hips anchored to the floor.
- If the neck begins to ache place the right hand behind the head (care must be taken not to pull the head forwards).

- Keep the shoulder-blades drawn down and the neck long.
- Keep the abdomen held in and flat.

Progression
- Reach a little higher up the leg ensuring that the abdominals are held flat.
- Place the supporting hand behind the head and lift the elbow off the floor.
- Place both hands behind the head.

Summary

- Contraction of TrA compresses and flattens the abdominal wall and reduces separation of RA.
- TrA co-contracts with the pelvic floor muscles.
- The aponeurosis from the three layers of muscle forms the rectus sheath.
- The aponeurosis, not the muscles, is cut during a caesarian section.
- The linea alba is formed by the joining of the aponeurosis of TrA and internal/external obliques from each side.
- The abdominal muscles are affected by relaxin which allows the rectus abdominis to stretch and separate.
- Rectus abdominis may lengthen by approximately 20cm and the waistline may increase by approximately 50cm.
- The muscles begin to realign three to four days after delivery, but may take six weeks or longer to repair.
- Caesarian deliveries may experience more difficulty recruiting TrA.
- TrA strengthening will assist realignment of linea alba.
- Exercises in four-point kneeling should be postponed until after six weeks.
- Rectus abdominis should be tested for separation prior to the commencement of gravity-resisted exercises.
- Separation of less than two fingers indicates that strengthening work can commence.
- Rectus abdominis should be shortened and strengthened within its inner range.
- The muscles should not be allowed to dome during a curl-up.
- Correct head alignment is essential.
- Exercises for the oblique muscles can commence when RA has been shortened and realigned and TrA has regained some strength.
- Movements that stress the muscles or pull them further apart may jeopardise abdominal recovery. Abdominal care is essential.

THE PELVIC FLOOR

The structure of the pelvic floor

The pelvic floor is a muscular platform at the base of the pelvis. Formed by a combination of muscles and fascia it resembles a sling, attached to the walls of the pelvis from the pubic bone at the front to the coccyx at the back. It consists of two halves joined in the middle to allow the urethra, vagina and anus to pass through. Superficial muscles form a figure 8 around these openings. The pelvic floor comprises four layers:

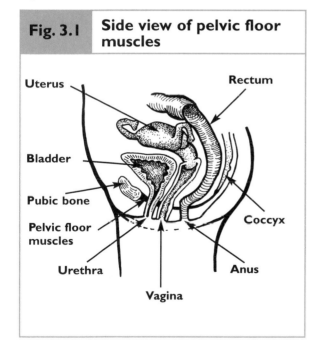

Fig. 3.1 Side view of pelvic floor muscles

- Uterus
- Rectum
- Bladder
- Pubic bone
- Coccyx
- Pelvic floor muscles
- Urethra
- Anus
- Vagina

1 A layer of fascia made of fibromuscular tissue consisting of collagen, elastin and smooth muscle fibres which surrounds and suspends the pelvic organs. This fascia provides limited support but requires the assistance of the pelvic floor muscles (PFM) when under pressure.

2 Levator ani muscle group consists of three muscles, formed in pairs, which attach in the middle and interconnect with the layers of fascia above and below. They form a muscular platform through which the urethra, vagina and anus pass.

3 The perineal membrane is made of collagen fascia and lies directly below the levator ani muscles. It provides support when the levator ani muscles relax.

4 Superficial muscles consist of three small muscles arranged in a figure of 8 around the openings. They offer minimal assistance to the continence mechanism and a small amount of support.

Slow- and fast-twitch muscle fibres

Skeletal muscle contains both slow- and fast-twitch muscle fibres and the PFM are no exception. The slow-twitch fibres work

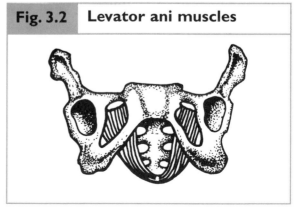

Fig. 3.2 Levator ani muscles

constantly at a low level to support the pelvic organs and maintain continence. They are slow to fatigue. The fast-twitch fibres have the ability to produce immediate strong contractions around the bladder neck and urethra to counteract sudden rises in intra-abdominal pressure – the cough reflex. These muscle fibres are quick to fatigue. Both types are found in the levator ani muscles (Jozwik and Jozwik 1998). The normal pattern of recruitment begins with slow-twitch fibres followed by fast, as additional strength is required, but during coughing or sneezing this pattern is reversed (Johnson 2001).

Fig. 3.3	**Superficial muscles of the pelvic floor**

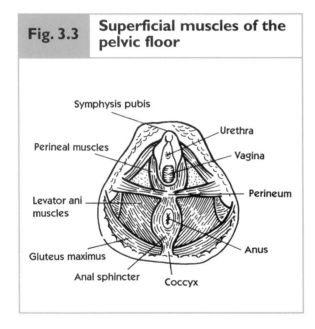

Symphysis pubis

Urethra

Perineal muscles

Vagina

Perineum

Levator ani muscles

Anus

Gluteus maximus

Anal sphincter

Coccyx

Functions of the pelvic floor

- To support the organs of the pelvis (bladder, uterus and bowel) and maintain their optimum angle.
- To resist sudden rises in intra-abdominal pressure such as coughing, sneezing, lifting and straining.
- To play a significant role in the continence mechanism.

- To help rotate the baby's head during delivery.
- To increase sexual satisfaction.
- To co-activate with TrA to assist pelvic-spinal stability.
- To have an inhibitory effect on bladder activity.

Mechanics of continence

During sudden rises in intra-abdominal pressure, the PFM contract and lift the bladder neck higher into the abdominal cavity. This reinforces urethral closure pressure and prevents urine escaping (Sapsford et al. 1998). Studies by King et al. (1998) suggests that pregnancy and birth affect bladder neck mobility and PFM exercises elevate the bladder neck and assist in the continence mechanism.

Changes to the pelvic floor during pregnancy

Increased levels of relaxin produced during pregnancy are believed to affect the two layers of fascia which encase levator ani, and weaken the whole support mechanism. Research suggests that it is pregnancy, rather than childbirth itself, which has the greatest effect on the PFM, with 64 per cent of women developing incontinence symptoms during this time (Charelli and Campbell 1997). It is thought that one of the contributory factors may be increased mobility in the bladder neck, decreasing support and reducing the closing pressure, creating leaks.

Collagen make-up determines the strength of the PFM, therefore a woman who experiences severe stretch marks, or is hypermobile is very likely to have problems with her PFM.

Additionally the uterus, which is not a fixed organ, is suspended by ligaments and therefore relies on the pelvic floor for the majority of its support. The increasing weight of the pregnant uterus places additional and progressive pressure on the weakening pelvic floor, putting it severely at risk. It is not uncommon for women to suffer stress incontinence (*see* page 40) in late pregnancy because of these changes.

Effects of labour and delivery on the pelvic floor

During labour and delivery the Levator ani muscles must relax to allow the baby to descend down the birth canal. It provides a pathway to guide the baby's head downwards, and strong muscles will help the baby to turn. Although relaxin has increased its elasticity, the PFM and superficial perineum still have a tremendous amount of stretching to do in the second stage of labour as the outlet area is forced open. If the baby's progress down the birth canal is very quick, and the perineum has insufficient time to stretch adequately, or the perineum and PFM lack sufficient elasticity to stretch over the baby's head, they may tear.

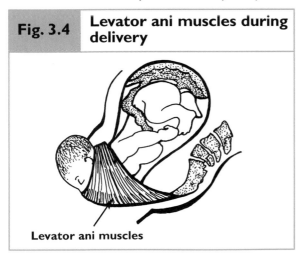

Fig. 3.4 Levator ani muscles during delivery

Levator ani muscles

Trauma to the perineum may occur through tearing, episiotomy, swelling or bruising.

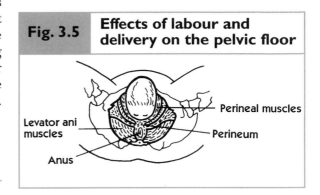

Fig. 3.5 Effects of labour and delivery on the pelvic floor

Levator ani muscles

Anus

Perineal muscles

Perineum

Episiotomy

An episiotomy is an incision in the perineum to enlarge the vaginal opening. It is performed to avoid excessive tearing or to speed up the delivery, usually if the baby is distressed. An episiotomy is also used in conjunction with an assisted delivery such as forceps, as it allows more space for the use of instruments in the vagina.

Stitches

If the perineum has been cut in an episiotomy, or a tear continues to bleed, it will be repaired with stitches. Healing usually occurs within 10 days, but it may take up to six weeks for stitches to dissolve.

Caesarean delivery

Many women who deliver by caesarean section do not appreciate the need to continue PFM exercises. Although these muscles have not experienced the excessive stretching and trauma of a vaginal delivery, relaxin has still increased its elasticity and the muscles have supported the growing baby for nine months.

As previously mentioned, studies have indicated that it is pregnancy rather than labour that is the cause of stress incontinence, so the case for pelvic floor exercises is still strong regardless of the type of delivery.

Stress incontinence

Stress incontinence is the involuntary loss of urine during physical exertion, i.e. coughing, sneezing, straining, lifting or jumping. It is not uncommon after childbirth and is often associated with:

- Overstretching of one or more of the muscle layers, decreasing organ support.
- Increased bladder neck mobility.
- Overstretching of the pudendal nerve responsible for activating the PFM. Damage to this nerve will affect the ability of the muscle to contract. This is usually associated with a difficult labour, especially forceps delivery.
- Forceps deliveries – Kessel et al. (2001) suggest a tenfold increase.

Unfortunately many women believe it is a natural consequence of having children and accept the condition. If exercises are not commenced or professional advice not sought the muscles will deteriorate and increase the risk of short- and long-term complications. A regular programme of correctly performed PFM exercises may resolve this problem; if not, referral to a physiotherapist specialising in women's health may be necessary.

Pelvic floor repair

The perineum may feel very sore and uncomfortable for many days after delivery, and it may be difficult to find a comfortable sitting position. The idea of exercising that area may cause concern about damaging it further. Despite apprehensions, gentle exercise will actually promote healing and aid recovery. During muscular contraction, blood flow to the area is increased, bringing with it nutrients for tissue repair and removing waste products. Exercises will reduce the pain and discomfort experienced from a swollen and tender perineum, and assist the edges of a cut/tear to close together.

When should pelvic floor exercises commence?

PFM exercises (PFME) should begin as soon as possible after the baby is born, ideally whilst still in the delivery room! If they are not undertaken the muscles will remain stretched and become further weakened with daily activities; recovery will then be much more difficult. Women who have never performed a PFME may experience difficulty in learning the process after delivery, as the muscles are stretched and weak and the response to their contractions so poor that nothing at all is felt. Recent research (Sapsford et al. 2001) suggest that PFM co-contract with TrA and vice versa. This is a useful starting point for women who find these exercises difficult or uncomfortable to do but should not be relied on as the only method of training. PFME must still be performed.

Effective teaching

It is advisable to spend time explaining the structure and function of the PFM before exercises are commenced. Launching straight into the exercises with no prior information will reduce their effectiveness. Whilst women will have been instructed to do these exercises after the birth, they may not be aware of their importance. A sore perineum may have discouraged commencement of the exercises or women may just have forgotten to do them. Basic, user-friendly language, appropriate to the individual or group, is essential to focus attention on the position and functions of these muscles. To clarify their supportive role, a model of a pelvis can be used, with both hands cupped underneath, to represent the muscles. Women must understand exactly what it is they are trying to do, particularly as nothing can be seen to be happening, and a clear explanation will help to build a better mental picture. A method of visualisation teaching is to imagine the pelvic floor as a lift, which tightens as the lift doors close and raises up as the lift rises to the first floor. They can be encouraged to try and lift to the second or even third floor and hold before lowering slowly down to the ground floor.

Muscle location and strength testing

Stopping the flow of urine mid-stream will give a good indication of PFM strength and is a good method of locating the correct muscles. However, it is essential that this method is used only as a test and not repeated regularly; stopping and starting the flow may create problems with the contraction/relaxation relationship of the bladder and PFM. Some women may not have the strength to stop or even slow down the flow of urine with a full bladder. Attempting to work weakened muscles in this way can cause additional stress, loss of control and great anxiety. On the few occasions when this test is undertaken, it is essential to allow sufficient time to completely empty the bladder. Another approach may be to suggest they grip their partner's penis during intercourse may be a preferable method, it this may be met with mixed reactions at the time! It

is particularly helpful if feedback is available! Approaches to teaching will vary and selection of the most appropriate method will depend on the client/group and the instructor's rapport with them.

Language

Clear, frank language is crucial. Avoiding essential terminology because of fear of embarrassment is unhelpful and will be counter-productive. Variations include:

- stopping the flow of urine/passing water/ having a pee/wee;
- stopping yourself passing/breaking wind;
- tightening/pulling up/in the vagina;
- gripping the penis/willy.

Re-educating the pelvic floor

Selecting an appropriate position to retrain the PFM is crucial in the early postnatal weeks to achieve a satisfactory muscular response. More success should initially be achieved in side or back lying positions as this reduces the load on the PFM, progressing to seated positions once strength has been regained. Exercises should be performed a few at a time, but frequently throughout the day. Initially it may be easier to begin with the quick exercise (*see* page 42), pausing briefly in between each contraction to avoid early fatigue. If this goes well introduce the slow exercise, holding the contraction for a few seconds initially and gradually increasing the length of hold. It is imperative to ensure that there is something left to release at the end rather than holding for longer and finding the contraction has already faded away. A controlled lowering should be practised. When coughing, sneezing or lifting, the pelvic floor should always be tightened to withstand the increased pressure. The quick exercise should still be practised as this will help to strengthen this reflex action.

Once control has been regained in a seated position, women should be encouraged to incorporate PFME into daily activities such as feeding the baby, nappy changing, lifting, carrying etc. Performing them in these functional positions is essential for improvement, but it is important that correct body alignment is practised; research suggests that exercises are more beneficial when a neutral spine position is adopted (Sapsford et al. 2001). It is important to concentrate to achieve the best quality performance and the exercise should be repeated several times on each occasion. Both the slow and the quick contractions should be practised as they each fulfil a different purpose.

Purpose of slow and fast exercises

Slow PFME will improve the tone of the muscle; this maintains the bladder neck at its optimum angle so that when intra-abdominal pressure increases, the fast PFM can contract to prevent urine loss. If the levator ani has low muscle tone it becomes flaccid and cannot support the bladder neck. When the fast PFM are required to prevent leakage, no matter how strong this reflex action is, if the bladder neck is not correctly aligned the fast PFM cannot prevent the loss of urine. Both types must be practised as they work together to provide optimum support.

Slow pelvic floor exercise

Purpose: to strengthen the slow-twitch muscles of the pelvic floor to provide support to the pelvic organs.

Preparation
In any position – lying, standing or sitting – with the feet slightly apart.

Action
- Draw up and tighten the muscles around the back and front passages.
- Lift them up inside you.
- Hold for a few seconds, continuing to breathe.
- Release and lower with control.
- Repeat 10 times.

NB If the contraction fails after a few seconds and there is nothing left to release, duration of hold should be shortened.

Technique tips
- Keep breathing throughout.
- Avoid tightening the buttock muscles.

Caution: Do not perform this exercise whilst passing urine.

Quick pelvic floor exercise

Purpose: to strengthen the fast-twitch muscle fibres of the pelvic floor (to prevent urine leakage).

Preparation
As for the slow exercise.

Action
- Tighten and lift the whole of the pelvic floor up in one quick contraction.
- Hold for a count of one.
- Release with control.
- Aim to repeat 10 times.*

Technique tips
- Keep breathing throughout.
- Avoid tightening the buttock muscles.

- Keep the body relaxed throughout – avoid bracing.

* The aim of this exercise is to try and perform each contraction with the same speed and strength as the first. Initially this will be very difficult to do as the fast-twitch muscle fibres will fatigue very quickly.

Effective training methods

There is no limit to the number of PFMEs to perform daily, providing the muscles are not fatigued. They should be realistic to the individual and performed with thought and as much accuracy as possible. Research indicates that effective training needs to be intensive and specific, and carried out for at least eight weeks. An increase in strength can be achieved by performing three blocks of exercise daily which should aim to include 10 slow (progressing towards 10 sec hold) and 10 quick repetitions on each occasion (Morkved and Bo 1996).

In the first 6–8 weeks after delivery, improvements in PFM strength are mainly attributed to recovery of the pudendal nerve supply which may have been damaged/stretched during labour and delivery. Once these neural connections have been made the muscles can begin to respond to training. Research suggests that it takes at least 300 repetitions before the muscle starts to register the contraction, so once they have been 'reconnected' the strengthening programme can begin. Without sounding too discouraging, it takes 30,000 repetitions of a muscle in the same position for it to respond autonomically.

As with any muscle training programme, it is essential to overload the muscle to make it work harder than usual in order that adaptations can occur. This can be done by lengthening the hold of the slow contraction, increasing the number of repetitions, or reducing the rest intervals between contractions. All methods of progression introduced at the same time will not produce good results – choose one at a time.

For how long should the exercises be continued?

Exercises for the pelvic floor should be continued for life! Unfortunately, it is around the three-month mark that many women stop doing PFME – if no problems have been experienced. They have noticed an improvement (identified earlier as nerve repair) and feel the muscles have recovered but strength has not been regained. To maintain improvement, this exercise must be carried out continuously on a regular basis – if exercises stop, the muscles start to weaken in 4–6 weeks! Time spent learning to do them correctly and effectively now will enable them to be incorporated into their new lifestyle and remain as an essential daily undertaking.

Problems with performing pelvic floor exercises

- There is a tendency to hold the breath, particularly with the fast PFME. This should be discouraged as it increases blood pressure.
- The gluteal muscles are often tightened whilst attempting a contraction resulting in a pelvic tilt – sometimes at the expense of the PFM.
- Whilst the TrA will naturally tighten when the PFM contract, engagement of RA should be avoided as this braces the abdomen.
- Sitting with legs crossed is likely to engage the adductor and gluteal muscles. A relaxed position with feet hip-width apart is recommended.

Exercise and the pelvic floor

Providing the PFM are being exercised correctly and sufficiently, physical activity can recommence after a satisfactory postnatal check-up. Activities causing obvious stress to the PFM must be avoided, e.g. trampolining, high-impact aerobics and strength training, until strength has been regained and ligament laxity reduced. Studio resistance classes should be avoided if inexperienced, and participation only permitted using low weights. TrA strength is vital to stabilise and support these activities, so if they are weak RA will override them and this may increase pressure on the PFM as IAP rises. Studio cycling, whilst low-impact, may not be particularly comfortable with a sore perineum. Jogging is a popular postnatal activity, selected for its convenience, but is often undertaken by inexperienced runners, unfamiliar with correct style. An elevated running style is inappropriate; in addition to feeling most uncomfortable, it may jeopardise PFM recovery. Jogging with minimal vertical action is recommended after 12 weeks.

Abdominal exercises

Any type of abdominal work should always be preceded by contraction of the TrA. This will co-activate the PFM and help to maintain IAP. If this does not occur, particularly during vigorous, resisted abdominal work, increased pressure will be exerted on both the aforementioned musculatures and recovery jeopardised. The technique of drawing navel to spine prior to any movement should be emphasised and practised until it becomes automatic.

Summary

- The PF is a muscular platform at the base of the pelvis.
- It has two layers of muscle and two layers of fibrous tissue.
- Pregnancy has the greatest effect on PFM strength.
- Women who deliver by caesarian section still need to strengthen their PFM.
- PFME will speed up recovery of damaged tissue and reduce swelling.
- Stress incontinence is not uncommon after childbirth.
- PFME can help to control stress incontinence.
- Retraining should commence in positions of low resistance and progress to more functional positions.
- Perform fast and slow exercises.
- Recovery in the first 6–8 weeks is attributed to pudendal nerve repair.
- A strength programme should commence after this time.
- PFME should not be performed while passing urine.
- Movements that cause impact or increased pressure on the PFM should be avoided until strength has been regained.
- The PFM co-contract with TrA.
- Exercising TrA will increase PFM strength.

THE BREASTS

Structure

The breasts comprise glandular tissue, fibrous tissue and fat, the latter determining their size and shape. They have no muscle attachment and are held in place by ligaments. The breasts lie directly above the pectoral muscles which play a small supporting role.

Pregnancy changes

The breasts increase in size from the early months of pregnancy due to the production of pregnancy hormones. Oestrogen allows fat to be deposited and, together with relaxin, stimulates tissue growth. Progesterone develops the milk-producing cells. Total breast weight may increase to approximately 800 g. This large increase in size together with the effects of the hormone relaxin on the ligaments and fibrous tissue of the breast (*see* Chapter 1) leads to stretching and possibly sagging of the breast tissues. Wearing a supportive bra during pregnancy will help to prevent excessive drooping as will strengthening exercises for the pectoral muscles. A fourth hormone, prolactin, stimulates the production of colostrum, a yellowish fluid that leaks from the nipple and contains important nutrients for baby's first feeds.

Postnatal changes

For the first few days after delivery the breasts continue to produce colostrum as they did during pregnancy. Colostrum contains protein and sugar but no fat, and is rich in antibodies that the baby needs to develop immunity. Milk production commences when the level of oestrogen has fallen allowing the level of prolactin to rise. If a general anaesthetic has been administered this may take a little longer.

Engorgement

When the milk comes in, on about day three or four after delivery, the breasts become very hot, swollen and hard. This is called engorgement. It is due to an increased blood supply and retention of fluid in the breasts (oedema) causing swelling. Engorgement is reduced as the baby begins to suck and this stimulates the continued production of prolactin. If breastfeeding is not commenced, prolactin levels will decrease and engorgement slowly reduces.

Hormonal changes due to breastfeeding

Oestrogen

As prolactin rises, to support lactation, oestrogen falls. Low oestrogen levels prevent the menstrual cycle returning immediately, and although it does not give complete protection against conception, it is a method of spacing pregnancies!

Suppressed ovarian function does incur several physiological changes that are similar to those of the menopause (Cunningham et al. 1997). These include hot flushes, night sweats, reduced vaginal secretions and reduced emotional stability. The most dramatic side-effect however, is the quick and significant loss of bone mineral content which averages about 5 per cent during the first three months (Drinkwater and Chestnut 1991). This is because oestrogen is the essential element needed for maintaining bone density. It works in three key ways:

- Maintains the correct balance of bone formation and resorption.
- Helps the body absorb calcium from the intestines.
- Reduces calcium loss through the kidneys.

The absence of oestrogen has a much greater effect on bone mass than exercise and calcium intake; if the latter two help bone by a factor of 2, then oestrogen helps bone by a factor of 10 (Otis and Goldingay 2000). Despite this, breastfeeding women are still recommended to take at least 1500 mg of calcium a day and may also need to supplement vitamin D as this facilitates calcium absorption. (Outdoor walking should be encouraged as sunlight provides a natural source of vitamin D.)

Prolactin

Prolactin levels vary during the first three months after delivery and are determined by the frequency of suckling:

- During the first week they are high, but only slightly increase with suckling.
- Between 2–12 weeks, levels increase 2–3 times and regular suckling incurs a further 10–20-fold increase.
- After three months, baseline prolactin levels are similar to those of non-lactating women and these do not rise significantly with suckling (Blackburn 2003). Reduction of prolactin levels at this time allows oestrogen

to rise and the consequential return of the menstrual cycle.

Exercise and bone mineral loss

Unfortunately, exercising does not appear to alter the rate of bone mineral loss in breastfeeding women (Clapp 1998) but regular weight-bearing activities and resistance training are strongly recommended to increase muscle mass and to support weakened structures.

Postural changes

The increased size and weight of the breasts pull the spine forwards; this, together with the positions often adopted for feeding, may cause stress and discomfort to the cervical and thoracic spine as it is pulled out of alignment. Correct posture should be adopted at all times, with particular emphasis on an extended, upright spine with the shoulders down and back (*see* Chapter 1). Women who were previously quite small-chested may feel self-conscious about their new development but should be encouraged to keep the chest lifted to maintain correct postural alignment. Although information is given to new mothers regarding positions for feeding, they are not always practical to adopt, especially if baby is particularly fractious or having problems latching on to the breast. Poor feeding positions will increase the stress to the spine and create tension and aching in the neck and shoulders, which, if repeated on a regular basis, may cause a great deal of discomfort. The correct posture for feeding is discussed in the Appendix.

Exercise and breastfeeding

Exercise and milk production

When exercise commences after the postnatal check-up, care should be taken not to do too much too soon. Dehydration and fatigue as a result of high intensity workouts may reduce the amount of milk available for the next feed. There has been considerable concern, in the past, that the combination of exercise and breastfeeding may reduce the quality and quantity of milk. These concerns relate to the levels of lactic acid in breast milk, which appear to give the milk a sour taste following intense aerobic activity. Studies suggest that changes in lactate levels of maternal blood or breastmilk occur only when exercise intensity is raised above the aerobic threshold (Quinn and Carey 1997). However, some babies become unsettled and don't feed well following a moderate intensity exercise session, so it would seem there are other factors involved here. Possible explanations may relate to maternal odour, sweat and degree of relaxation.

Intake and exercise performance

Research indicates that women who exercise and breastfeed naturally increase their calorie intake (Dewey et al. 1994) but frequently do not increase fluid intake sufficiently. Low fluid intake is directly associated with poor performance in both exercise and breastfeeding and a minimum of 4 litres per day is recommended! As a guide, women can determine how hydrated they are by checking the colour of their urine – the clearer the urine the better hydrated.

Breastfeeding and weight loss

The body needs an extra 600 calories per day to ensure an adequate supply of milk, and appetite generally increases in response to this. Fat utilisation increases during breastfeeding and this will assist weight loss, particularly if combined with moderate exercise and sensible eating. Drastic dieting or repeated sessions of very intense exercise may significantly reduce milk quality and production, or it may cease completely.

Exercise considerations

Feed before exercising

It is essential to feed or express milk before exercising to decrease the load and reduce leakage. Large, full breasts will feel uncomfortable if squeezed or bumped and vigorous, large-range arm movements may promote milk flow. However, this cannot always be avoided and a small amount of milk loss is not uncommon during exercise.

Range of movement

The range of movement for some arm exercises may have to be reduced to maintain comfort. Elbow alignment may be difficult to maintain and consideration should be given to the fact that breast tissue also extends into the armpit. With the added concern of the lingering effects of relaxin, adaptations are essential – body positioning and joint alignment should not be compromised in the desire to achieve results. Movements should continue within the regular range until breastfeeding ceases.

Body positioning

For most women, the breasts may feel extremely uncomfortable when exercising in a prone position. For others, this position may be tolerated for short periods, providing feeding time is not imminent. Rolled-up towels placed above and below the breasts may reduce some of the pressure but this should be monitored as it may hyperextend the spine. Alternative positions or equipment should be used where possible, or commencement postponed until the prone position is comfortable. Inverted/ forward leaning positions or four-point kneeling may cause additional drag and discomfort to heavy breasts. Stretches for the pectoral muscles should be performed with the abdominals lightly held in and ribcage drawn down to prevent hyperextension.

What type of bra should be worn?

A good supporting bra is essential during exercise to prevent overstretching of the breast tissue. Whilst a nursing bra is very convenient for feeding it does not provide sufficiently adequate support for exercising. A sports bra is strongly recommended as it is designed to absorb shock and reduce the bounce of the breasts during physical activity (this could be worn over the top of a nursing bra if necessary). Wide shoulder straps help to distribute the weight across the shoulders more evenly and this will help prevent neck, shoulder, and upper back pain. Tight-fitting, elasticated crop tops, that compress the breasts into the chest wall, may constrict the milk ducts and lead to mastitis.

Summary

- Prolactin rises to support lactation, and oestrogen falls.
- Reduced oestrogen causes significant bone mineral loss.
- Calcium intake should be increased to 1500 mg per day.
- Regular weight-bearing exercise is essential to increase muscle mass and support weakening bones.
- Large breasts will affect posture and may stress the spine.
- Poor posture and feeding positions may cause tension and aching in the upper back, shoulders and neck.
- Moderate-intensity exercise does not affect the quality and quantity of breastmilk.
- High-intensity exercise may reduce the amount of milk available for the next feed.
- An extra 600 calories per day are required to maintain an adequate supply of milk.
- Body weight may not return to normal until breastfeeding has ceased.
- A regular and plentiful intake of fluids is essential to avoid dehydration.
- Baby should be fed before exercise commences to reduce the weight of the breasts and decrease the possibility of milk loss.
- Vigorous arm movements may cause the breasts to leak.
- The range of movement for upper body work may have to be reduced.
- Alternative exercising positions may be necessary.
- A good supporting bra is essential.

POSTNATAL COMPLICATIONS

Joint problems

The pelvis

The symphysis pubis and sacroiliac joints are very closely related and a problem experienced in one area is generally consistent with misalignment of the whole pelvis (*see* Chapter 1).

Symphysis pubis pain

This joint at the front of the pelvis, where the two pubic bones meet, is extremely vulnerable during pregnancy. Increased laxity, caused by raised levels of relaxin on the supporting ligaments, together with pressure from the baby, enables the symphysis pubis to widen. It is considered normal for the gap between the two bones to increase from the non-pregnant 4 mm to approximately 9 mm. Post-delivery, this gap will begin to decrease within days, although the supporting ligaments will take much longer to provide full stability (*see* Chapter 1). The degree of pain experienced, however, is not indicative of the width of the separation; pain may occur in this area without excessive widening taking place. It is often associated with increased movement of one or both of the sacroiliac joints which then puts additional strain on the symphysis pubis. This condition is known as Symphysis Pubis Dysfunction (SPD). Excessive widening (1 cm or more), sometimes with the two bones being slightly out of alignment, is known as Diastasis Symphysis Pubis (DSP). This is a more serious condition and fortunately less common than SPD (*see* Appendix for details of support group).

What are the symptoms?

Mild to severe pain in the area of the pubis and groin, radiating down the inside of the leg. It may be extremely painful to touch. This may intensify when walking, particularly upstairs, turning over in bed and opening the legs to get in and out of the car. In severe cases a grinding or clicking sound may be heard each time the joint is moved and it may become increasingly difficult to remain mobile.

Sacroiliac pain

Pain in the sacroiliac joint can be attributed to a couple of possible changes.

- Increased joint laxity allowing greater movement in one or both joints.
- The two joint surfaces becoming stuck and producing a locked joint as opposed to a moving joint.

What are the symptoms?

Mild to severe pain around the joint, radiating across the buttock and up into the lumbar spine. Pain in the buttocks and down the back of the leg may be the result of sacroiliac misalignment causing pressure on the sciatic nerve, which runs immediately behind the sacroiliac joint. Discomfort or pain may also be felt in the symphysis pubis.

Are these postnatal conditions?

The onset of symphysis pubis and sacroiliac pain may occur during or after pregnancy. Some conditions may rectify themselves after the birth or continue into the postnatal period, others may be caused by the passage of the baby through the pelvis during delivery, increasing the pressure on the lax joints. Occasionally problems may occur as a result of the lithotomy position, particularly if the legs were not placed in, or removed from the stirrups simultaneously. This is more likely to occur with an epidural, when painful separation of the legs is masked by the anaesthetic.

What can be done to help?

Reduce weight-bearing activities and avoid standing on one leg or distributing the weight unevenly (hoovering is particularly inappropriate!). Avoid straddle movements which take the legs apart, and try to keep the knees and feet together when turning over in bed and getting into and out of the car. Correct standing posture should be practised at all times with particular attention to back and abdominal care when meeting the numerous demands of a new baby (*see* Chapters 1 and 2). TrA and pelvic floor exercises are essential to assist stabilisation of the pelvis (*see* Chapters 2 and 3) together with low-resistance gluteal work, i.e. pelvic tilting with additional gluteal squeeze. Progressing from the pelvic tilt into bridge may increase pressure through the joint if taken too high.

Force closure

To assist stabilisation of these joints, Vleeming (1990) recommends working the muscles that lie in the oblique sling to create additional force to close it. The posterior oblique sling refers to latissimus dorsi and opposing gluteus maximus which, when co-contracted, will assist with stabilisation of the sacroiliac joint (*see* kneeling, arm & leg raise exercise, page 22). Tension created in the thoracolumbar fascia, as a result of the combined contraction, increases compression in the sacroiliac joints and assists stabilisation. The anterior oblique sling refers to internal/external obliques, TrA and opposing adductors, which when contracted will assist

with stabilisation of the symphysis pubis (*see* scissor arms with leg slide, page 19 and bridge with heel raise, page 106). It is important to remember that individuals will differ and not all exercises will be suitable.

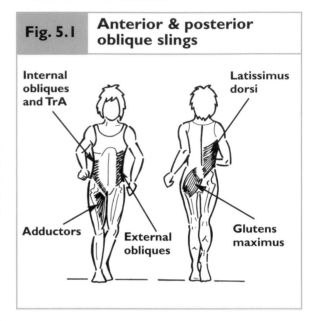

Fig. 5.1 Anterior & posterior oblique slings

Internal obliques and TrA

Latissimus dorsi

Adductors

External obliques

Glutens maximus

Exercise and symphysis pubis/sacroiliac pain

Those able to participate in physical activity should consider the following:

- Exercises for the adductor muscles. Pain in the symphysis pubis may be experienced with this movement due to the attachment of the adductor muscles to the pubic bone itself. When they contract the muscles pull on the pubic bone as the leg is drawn in.
- Exercises for the abductor muscles. This may cause pain or discomfort either to the symphysis pubis or the sacroiliac joints due to pelvic misalignment.
- Cross-trainers and steppers may aggravate a problem due to the repeated shift of body weight from one foot to the other over a prolonged period of time.

- Sidesteps and knee bends should not be taken too wide.
- Movements performed on one leg (some yoga postures) may increase the stress on the supporting side due to pelvic misalignment.
- Rocking the hips excessively from side to side in any movement, particularly when walking quickly, should be avoided.
- Breaststroke leg action whilst swimming may stress the symphysis pubis.
- Sitting cross-legged and similar yoga postures may be uncomfortable.

It should be considered that women attending an exercise session may not present with these problems initially, and may actually experience this pain for the first time during the session. Symphysis pubis and/or sacroiliac pain may be the source of much discomfort and aggravation and if symptoms persist women should be encouraged to seek the advice of a physiotherapist specialising in women's health.

Damaged coccyx

The coccyx is joined to the sacrum at the sacrococcygeal joint, which allows movement of the coccyx during delivery. The coccyx may bruise or occasionally fracture if it is pushed backwards during the second stage of labour. The resulting pain can be severe and incapacitating and will make sitting extremely difficult.

What can be done to help?

Sitting, particularly on hard surfaces, will be impossible, and alternative positions, such as side lying, may need to be found for feeding. Relief may be gained from sitting on an inflatable or valley cushion (*see* Appendix) to reduce pressure on the coccyx. A child's rubber ring is particularly helpful to sit on in the bath.

It is important to keep all pressure off the coccyx to allow it to heal.

Exercise and a damaged coccyx

Floorwork will pose the greatest difficulties. It may be extremely uncomfortable, or even impossible, to lie supine in neutral alignment and it may be necessary to tilt the pelvis posteriorly, to pull the coccyx forward and reduce pressure on the area. Seated floor positions may need to be adapted (i.e. hamstring/adductor stretches) and any seated exercise that involves rolling off the sit bones should be eliminated from the programme. The seated recumbent bike may also be inappropriate.

The knee

Softening of the articular cartilage of the patella may sometimes occur during pregnancy as a result of the effects of increased relaxin on collagen tissue. Widening of the pelvis may increase the Q-angle of the femur at the knee joint and pull the patella out of alignment. Weight gain and altered posture will also increase the stress to the knee joint. Pain or aching will be felt in the front of the knee when it is flexed (sitting, squatting, standing up) and is accentuated when walking downstairs. The increased need to bend, squat or kneel down while caring for a baby may exacerbate this condition.

Exercise and knee pain

All activities involve knee flexion at some stage, and it would be impossible to completely eliminate the action. However, obvious knee flexion, i.e. step training or cycling, should be avoided and alternative exercises selected.

Alternatives may need to be found for kneeling floorwork exercises, to reduce the pressure on the joint. Increasing the strength of the quadriceps, particularly vastus medialis, will be helpful to provide support around the knee joint (*see* leg extension, page 105).

Backache

This is a very common postnatal complaint experienced by a large percentage of women, many of whom were not affected during pregnancy. The lingering effects of relaxin on spinal stability continue into the postnatal period and the increased size of the breasts and poor feeding positions place further stresses on the thoracic and cervical areas. Weak, stretched, abdominal muscles are not able to support the spine sufficiently and this problem is compounded by the constant bending and lifting necessary for everyday babycare. Discomfort may be experienced in all areas of the spine although the lumbar region tends to suffer most. Women who had epidurals may experience added discomfort but there is no evidence to suggest that epidurals themselves cause backache. It is more likely that poor body alignment was adopted during delivery and the anaesthetic masked the discomfort of the incorrect position. Bruising from the epidural site may be felt for several weeks. Tiredness and fatigue associated with a new baby should also be considered as a contributory factor to the general aches and pains frequently experienced.

What can be done to help?

Postural correction plays an essential role in postnatal back care. Body positions should be carefully revised for standing and sitting, particularly during feeding, and correct techniques adopted for lifting and carrying baby (*see* Chapter 1 and Appendix). Strengthening exercises for the TrA (*see* pages 16–26) are vital, as these muscles compress the abdomen towards the spine to provide support and stability. Pelvic floor muscle exercises are also recommended. Stretching exercises for the trapezius, latissimus dorsi, gluteals, hamstrings, hip flexors and piriformis may help to release unwanted tension (*see* Chapters 8 and 9). Women should be encouraged to rest as much as possible during the day and adopt good postural positions that enable the spine to release, i.e. lying supine on a firm surface with legs lifted to 90 degrees and supported on a chair.

Separation of the abdominal muscles (diastasis recti)

During pregnancy the abdominal muscles undergo a tremendous amount of stretching, facilitated by the increased production of relaxin. The two bands of recti muscles, which were previously parallel, stretch away from the midline to allow space for the growing uterus. This is reported to occur in 66 per cent of women during the third trimester of pregnancy (Boissonault 1988). The size of the separation can vary between a small gap measuring 2–3 cm wide and 12–15 cm long, to a larger gap of 12–20 cm wide which may extend almost the length of the recti muscles. Due to the structure of the musculature, the greatest point of separation is usually around the area of the umbilicus, which forms a crossroads between linea alba and the lowest tendinous inscription.

Causes of large separation

Women with a narrow pelvis who carried their baby 'all at the front' are most at risk, as are those who experienced multiple births. Close pregnancies may also be a contributory factor as the muscles are not given adequate time and/or exercise to repair and realign before pregnancy recurs. Women who undertake an activity during pregnancy which specifically stretches or stresses the abdominal muscles are also at risk; activities such as wind-surfing and strong resisted abdominal exercises, particularly for the oblique muscles, are inappropriate. A sedentary lifestyle is not the answer, however, as women with extremely weak abdominal muscles may not have sufficient strength for the muscles to realign. Separation may occur during the second stage of labour when intra-abdominal pressure increases, causing the uterus to push outwards against the abdominal wall. Poor postnatal abdominal care when sitting up or lying down will increase the pressure on the muscles, as will abdominal strengthening exercises performed with poor technique. It is essential to draw the abdominals in prior to movement, to prevent the abdomen pushing up between the ridges of widened muscle and forcing the two sides further apart (*see* doming, p. 28).

How will you know this has happened?

Perform the 'rec check' test for the abdominals outlined on page 27 to determine the width of the separation. Due to the structure of the musculature, everyone will have a gap of some degree between the muscle bands. Gross separation is classified as a gap of more than two fingers (approx. 3 cm) three days post-delivery. This may be felt a few centimetres above and below the umbilicus or it may just be present below the umbilicus. In more severe cases it may involve the majority of the linea alba and extend from the breastbone to the pubis.

When could you expect this to repair?

For the majority of women the width of the gap will reduce to two fingers or less by the time she has her postnatal check-up at around six weeks.

Separation of more than two fingers at this time does not necessarily indicate a permanent problem. If correct abdominal exercises are performed the muscles can be encouraged to shorten and realign further (see below). In cases of gross separation, the abdomen will remain distended and pendulous and may need surgical repair. In this case, lack of support from the abdominal muscles increases pressure on the vertebral discs when lifting and is likely to cause backache and possible injury. Repair involves stitching the two sides of the recti muscle together.

What can be done to help?

Re-education of abdominal posture is crucial at this time and women should be encouraged to be constantly aware of it in every position throughout the day. Drawing navel to spine is a simple exercise which can easily be integrated into daily activities. This will reduce the horizontal stretch of TrA and help to stabilise linea alba. Appropriate care of the abdominals during everyday activities is essential, particularly when getting up from lying down, when it is imperative that the body is rolled on to one side before sitting up, and reversed when lying down. Allowing the body to move straight up and down from this position places high demands on the abdominal muscles and delays recovery. When bending forwards for nappy changing the abdomen should be tightened to prevent it from hanging down and the muscles used for support on every occasion.

Exercise and diastasis recti

Abdominal hollowing to shorten and strengthen TrA should be commenced as soon as possible in a variety of positions. The prone lying position is particularly beneficial (*see* p. 17), although this may be unsuitable if breastfeeding. Four-point kneeling (box) position should not be adopted before six weeks (*see* p. 21) Whilst this is an excellent exercise after this time, it should be treated with caution if the abdomen is particularly pendulous as this may place additional stretch on the abdominal musculature. All the Level 1 TrA exercises in Chapter 2 are suitable and should be the initial focus for abdominal recovery. In addition, it is recommended that the supine and kneeling pelvic tilt (*see* pages 30 and 31) is also introduced to help reduce the vertical stretch on the recti muscles. Head and shoulder raising can be introduced at this stage but may need to commence with a pillow underneath the head to reduce the range of movement (*see* page 32). It is imperative that this exercise is performed with the correct technique and the height of the raise determined by the strength of the TrA muscles to keep the abdomen pulled in. Doming will occur if the head and shoulders are raised too high for the abdominals to maintain control. This must be avoided at all times. Once the maximum height of the curl has been ascertained, this position, just prior to doming, should be held for 2–3 seconds and the abdominals encouraged to draw in further. When this can be performed in a controlled manner, the range of movement can be increased by removing the pillow from behind the head. All exercises should be performed slowly and with control. Twisting curl-ups for the oblique muscles are contra-indicated if the abdominals have a separation of more than 3 cm (*see* Chapter 2).

Pelvic floor damage

The pelvic floor is composed of muscles, nerves and connective tissue; damage to any of these structures has implications for its function. Overstretching of one or more layers decreases organ support and causes the descent of the bladder neck, which reduces urethral closing pressure. Research suggests that the PFM have the ability to be trained providing weakness is not due to nerve damage or torn muscles. In such cases, stretch damage to the pudendal nerve, which lies within the PF musculature, reduces nerve connection to the muscle and affects the fast-twitch reflex action. This is known to cause urinary incontinence (Snooks et al. 1990). In such cases, referral to a physiotherapist specialising in women's health is essential. Pudendal nerve damage is usually associated with a difficult labour, especially forceps. Trauma to the perineum may occur through cutting or tearing.

Stress incontinence

Stress incontinence, as mentioned above, is the consequence of overstretched muscles or nerves within the PF musculature, which cannot withstand sudden rises in intra-abdominal pressure. This occurs when coughing, sneezing, laughing or during exertion such as lifting, jumping or running and results in a small leak of urine. This condition has a high incidence rate – 67 per cent of women at three months post-delivery (Marshall et al. 1996).

What can be done to help?

The success of PFM training is dependent on the individual's ability to identify and isolate the correct muscles, and this may prove to be the first hurdle. An intensive daily exercise programme should be devised, which includes both the fast- and slow-twitch muscle fibres (*see* Chapter 3). When commencing the programme it is important to begin in positions of lowest resistance first, i.e. side- or supine-lying, progressing to seated positions once success has been achieved. Start with the fast contraction, allowing a pause in between each repetition, and keep a record of how many can be performed with equal intensity (*see* page 41). If some success is gained with this then the slow exercise can be introduced as well, holding initially for a few seconds before gradually increasing the length of hold. Each contraction should aim to be of equal intensity and held for the same length of time – again, record-keeping is important. The aim is slowly to increase the hold up to 10 seconds, but this will take a great deal of time and effort to achieve. These blocks of exercise should be repeated as many times as possible throughout the day, every day. Evidence suggests that participation in a PFM exercise programme will cure up to 66 per cent of stress incontinence in postnatal women (Morkved and Bo 1996 and 2000). It is important to note that if a woman is experiencing stress incontinence and is having difficulty recruiting her PFM she should be referred to a physiotherapist specialising in women's health.

Exercise and stress incontinence

Activities that cause obvious impact to the pelvic floor should be avoided as this will exacerbate the condition, e.g. jumping, horse riding, trampolining and running (although this is dependent on the technique). Resistance training and vigorous abdominal work is not recommended as the rise in intra-abdominal pressure will further stress the weakened musculature. Pelvic floor exercises should be an integral part of the exercise regime and should be performed in sets of repetitions as with any other muscle group. It is important to note that the maintenance of good hydration levels is vital during exercise. Sufferers will probably prefer to avoid fluids prior to and during exercise for fear of an accident but dehydration increases the concentration of urine and further irritates the bladder.

Sore perineum

The perineum may be sore for some days or even weeks following delivery, and many women have difficulty finding a comfortable sitting position – making feeding more difficult. Discomfort may be experienced from bruising, haemorrhoids, or from an episiotomy or tear which has not repaired well, either because of poor stitching leading to lumpy scar tissue, or because of infection.

What can be done to help?

Pelvic floor exercises are invaluable to assist the healing process, although many women may be apprehensive about doing these if they are feeling uncomfortable. Pain may be more severe with the first contraction but should decrease with repetition as the swelling is reduced. Increased blood flow to the damaged tissue speeds up the healing process, removing waste products from the area and helping the edges of a cut or tear to close together. It is vital that the pelvic floor is contracted while coughing, sneezing or lifting to counter-brace the rise in intra-abdominal pressure.

Prolapse

A prolapse is the bulging of the bladder or rectum through the wall of the vagina, or the descent of the uterus into the vagina. These pelvic organs are held in position by ligaments and the PFM are sandwiched between layers of fascia, all of which are affected by relaxin. Further weakening or damage may occur during labour and/or delivery. Bulging of the bladder, to some degree, against the front wall of the vagina is the most common postnatal prolapse condition, although a prolapse of the rectum may sometimes occur. Uterine prolapse is more closely associated with the menopause when low levels of oestrogen decrease the elasticity of the vaginal walls. Other causes of a prolapse may be continuous heavy lifting (as in strength training), incorrect performance of PFME, i.e. bearing down rather than contracting and lifting up, chronic constipation or a chronic cough.

What are the symptoms of a prolapse?

A dragging sensation, or a feeling of something 'coming down' in the vagina which may be accompanied by backache. This feeling is experienced when standing and becomes progressive through the day. It appears to go when lying down. Stress incontinence may be present together with a frequent desire to urinate; this is due to an inability to completely empty the bladder because of the incorrect angle of the bladder neck (*see* page 42).

What can be done to help?

Pelvic floor exercises may delay or even prevent the need for surgery to repair a prolapse, as strong PFM will help to support the pelvic organs. It is important to maintain good hydration levels and avoid caffeine, which may irritate the bladder. To help the bladder to empty completely following urination, it may be helpful to stay seated on the toilet and rock the pelvis forward and back.

Exercise and prolapse

As with stress incontinence, high-impact activities are potentially damaging to the weakened ligaments and pelvic floor musculature and should be avoided if a prolapse is suspected. Resistance training should be reduced to very light weights and only gentle abdominal work attempted. PFM support is vital during such activities. Professional advice should be sought at the earliest opportunity.

Carpal tunnel syndrome

Carpal tunnel syndrome is caused by the compression of the median nerve as it passes through the narrow tunnel of bones in the wrist. Tingling and numbness is experienced in the thumb, index and middle fingers. It is often a condition of late pregnancy, associated with water retention, but it is not uncommon for it to develop after the birth. In extreme cases, sufferers may have difficulty caring for their baby. More severe symptoms of carpal tunnel syndrome have been experienced by women who breastfeed, and although symptoms often reduce a few days after weaning commences the problem may not resolve completely until breastfeeding has ceased. No physiological reason has been found yet for this.

What can be done to help?

Resting with the hands in an elevated position will assist with fluid drainage and may temporarily relieve discomfort. Finger and wrist mobility exercises whilst the hands are in this position are also recommended. Referral to a physiotherapist specialising in women's health may be necessary.

Exercise and carpal tunnel syndrome

Weight-bearing positions that require flexion of the wrist, e.g. four-point kneeling, may be extremely uncomfortable or in some cases impossible. The flexed angle of the wrist joint reduces blood flow to the fingers and gravity encourages a build-up of fluid. Correct wrist/forearm alignment is essential when using resistance equipment; lifts that require the arms to be in a downward position may be painful and induce loss of sensation in the fingers. Grip strength may also be affected, so care and attention should be given to the use of resistance equipment.

Mastitis

Mastitis is an inflammation of the breast that arises when milk is not emptied from the breast as quickly as it is produced. There are several possible causes of this:

- A blocked duct
- Incorrect positioning of the baby
- Pressure from the hands holding the breast to feed
- Tight seat belt
- Wearing a tight bra
- Cracked nipples leading to infection.

The breasts become red and lumpy and extremely painful, and women may feel feverish and quite ill. Unless this is treated quickly the breast may become infected and develop an abscess, which requires surgical removal and drainage.

Exercise following mastitis

Prone positions are most inappropriate due to the pressure on the breasts. An adapted front lying position with elbows supporting the upper body to keep the breasts off the floor is also unsuitable as it may stress the spine. Since the breast tissue extends into the armpit many arm movements may cause discomfort. A good supportive bra is essential but it should not be so tight that it constricts the breasts excessively.

Varicose veins

Varicose veins may occur during pregnancy, normally in the legs. They are caused by the relaxing effects of progesterone on the walls of the veins and the resulting inefficiency of the vein valves to close and secure a one-way flow of blood back to the heart. This causes the veins to swell and the legs to feel tired and heavy. After delivery there is often an improvement in the severity of this condition, although appropriate leg care should still be continued.

What can be done to help?

Avoid sitting with crossed legs or kneeling back on the heels as this will compress the veins and further reduce blood flow. Sitting with legs supported in a raised position whenever possible may reduce discomfort.

Exercise and varicose veins

Exercises that increase the blood flow through the calves are recommended, as the pumping action of the muscle will assist blood flow back to the heart. Walking is the ideal activity for its additional benefits, but standing ankle mobility and calf raises are equally helpful (*see* pages 93 and 104). Standing still should be avoided.

Haemorrhoids

Haemorrhoids are varicose veins in the anal passage. Relaxation of the smooth muscle tissue of the intestines during pregnancy results in increased fluid absorption and the slowing down of the passage of waste material through the gut. This often leads to constipation, and the consequent straining to move the bowels causes ballooning of the veins in and around the anus. Haemorrhoids may appear for the first time after delivery as a result of pushing in the second stage of labour and may cause extreme discomfort, e.g. itching around the anus and pain/bleeding when passing motions. Constipation will compound this problem.

What can be done to help?

The use of ice packs may ease the pain and reduce the swelling and frequent pelvic floor exercises will also be beneficial. The advice for constipation (see below) also applies here.

Constipation

Constipation is extremely common during the early postnatal weeks, probably due to:

- Fear of pain or tearing in the pelvic floor during excretion;
- Dehydration caused by loss of fluids in breast milk;
- Weak abdominals reducing intra-abdominal pressure;
- Inactivity – regular exercise helps prevent constipation;
- Insufficient fruit and fibre because of concerns over its effect on breast milk.

What can be done to help?

Gentle cardiovascular exercise such as walking is highly recommended as it increases the heart rate and promotes the circulation. Exercises to strengthen the TrA are essential (*see* Chapter 2). Women should be advised to drink plenty of water, increase their intake of fibre and avoid straining and holding the breath whilst on the toilet. Supporting the perineum with a pad of toilet paper, may be helpful during defecation, to prevent it bulging.

Emotional problems

Women may experience a variety of emotional problems following birth. These can occur immediately or develop slowly during the early months of motherhood.

- 'Baby blues' is a mild, transitory condition experienced in varying degrees by about 50 per cent of women. It generally commences a few days after delivery and lasts only a few days. Women feel emotional and upset, crying for seemingly trivial reasons, and may find it impossible to cheer up. Most mothers who have the blues feel very tired and lethargic; some may feel anxious and tense and many have difficulty sleeping.
- Postnatal depression may be mild, moderate or severe and can affect up to one in six new mothers. It can occur at any time within the first year but seems to be most common when the baby is between four and six months old. It may come on gradually over a period of time or start suddenly. Postnatal depression has many symptoms, often beginning in a similar way to baby blues but developing to more severe feelings of anxiety and stress. Some women suffer panic attacks and feel tense and irritable or become very anxious about their own and their baby's health. Most women suffering from postnatal depression feel guilty that they are not coping as well as they think they should.

What are the causes?

The birth of a baby is a deeply emotional time, bringing intense feelings of joy as well as overwhelming anxiety. Feelings of depression may be related to the sudden change in the level of the hormones after delivery. This is compounded by the physical demands of round-the-clock baby care and diminishing energy levels. Becoming a mother is a major role change; loss of independence and income, isolation and lack of adult conversation are all factors that contribute to emotional change at a time when a woman is already feeling exhausted and vulnerable.

What can be done to help?

Exercise can be extremely beneficial for women experiencing baby blues or mild postnatal depression, although their possible lack of motivation might prevent participation. A specific postnatal exercise class can be particularly helpful as it will provide sympathetic support from other new mums and an opportunity to share experiences and anxieties. Easy to follow, safe and effective exercise designed specifically to meet their postnatal needs will improve their physical endurance, reduce feelings of fatigue, and help rebuild self-confidence. Exercise of the appropriate intensity can also help with the dispersal of adrenalin, which builds up when the body is stressed and can improve mild to moderate depression. Encouragement and praise from the instructor is essential as well as increased sensitivity when correcting poor performance.

A period of structured relaxation is strongly recommended. This can help to ease muscle tension and rest the body. If anxiety levels are high, individuals may find it almost impossible to relax, but regular participation in a familiar relaxation procedure can be helpful over a period of time (*see* Chapter 14). Other strategies include taking time out, working out priorities and setting realistic, achievable goals. It is important to remember that postnatal depression is an illness and women need support from people who understand. Help and support is available (*see* Appendix for details).

Summary

- Pain in the symphysis pubis or sacroiliac joints may prevent exercise participation.
- Pain in the symphysis pubis is not indicative of the degree of separation.
- A damaged or bruised coccyx may prevent particular floor positions being adopted.
- Increased stress to the knee joint from the effects of pregnancy and babycare may induce knee problems.
- Correct posture can reduce backache.
- Exercises to strengthen TrA will help to realign rectus abdominis and reduce back pain.
- Resisted abdominal work should be performed with extreme caution if the muscles have separated more than two fingers. The abdomen should not be allowed to dome and exercises for the oblique muscles must be avoided.
- Damage to muscles, nerves and connective tissue of the pelvic floor has implications for its function.
- Pudendal nerve damage effects fast-twitch action and can lead to stress incontinence.
- An intensive daily programme is essential for pelvic floor recovery.
- Seated positions may be uncomfortable for a sore perineum.
- High-impact activities and strength training may increase the risk of a prolapse.
- Tingling and numbness in the fingers may limit the amount of weight-bearing exercises that can be performed. Grip strength may also be affected.
- Painful breasts following mastitis can reduce the range of movement in the upper body and prevent particular positions being adopted.
- Gentle cardiovascular exercise and increased fluid intake will help improve constipation and haemorrhoids.
- Exercise may improve mild postnatal depression.

ALL ABOUT EXERCISE

PART TWO

This section looks at different types of training methods and discusses their suitability for postnatal women and considerations for participation.

PHYSICAL FITNESS

What is physical fitness?

Physical fitness is a term that encompasses a number of components. An ideal exercise schedule should include all aspects of physical fitness so that demands are placed on all the body systems.

The components of fitness

Cardiovascular fitness is the ability of the heart, lungs and blood vessels to deliver oxygenated blood to the muscles to provide energy for them to work. The body benefits from cardiovascular fitness because there is sufficient oxygen to meet energy demands. Cardiovascular exercise also reduces the risk of heart disease. Additional benefits for a postnatal woman include increased circulation to improve the condition of varicose veins and assist with weight loss. Cardiovascular fitness is improved through activities such as walking, jogging, swimming, rowing, stepping, etc., often referred to as aerobic activities.

Muscle fitness includes *strength* and *endurance.*

Muscular *strength* is the amount of force a muscle, or group of muscles, can exert. It is important in everyday life to help with strenuous tasks such as lifting and carrying heavy shopping, moving furniture etc. Insufficient strength may prevent performance of a particular task or lead to injuries. Muscular strength varies enormously between individuals and training methods may range from gravity-resisted exercises to weight training in a gym

environment. It is inadvisable to train with heavy weights in the first six months after delivery (*see* Chapter 11).

Muscular *endurance* is the ability of the muscles to keep working over a period of time. Postnatally this is important for holding and carrying the baby, equipment, and shopping. Situations also arise where muscles have to endure more than they are really capable of, e.g. performing one-handed tasks while holding baby. This will result in muscle ache or may induce the assistance of other muscles if your body positioning is altered. Muscular endurance can be improved by using a light to moderate resistance and performing 12–20 repetitions. Body weight can be used against gravity to create the resistance, as in abdominal curls or press-ups, or with the use of equipment such as dumbbells, bands, body bars or resistance machines

Flexibility is the range of movement at a joint. It is necessary for everyday tasks that require a mobile body, e.g. bending forwards to put on shoes or reaching up to a high shelf, and postnatally a degree of flexibility will reduce the demands placed on the body when caring for baby. It is extremely important for the maintenance of correct posture and allows muscles to work within their optimum range (*see* Chapter 1). Flexibility is maintained and increased by stretching. While it is important, postnatally, to perform short-held stretches to maintain flexibility, it is inadvisable to stretch to increase flexibility through longer, more progressive stretches.

Motor fitness includes agility, co-ordination, balance and reaction time, requiring the brain to organise simultaneous bodily responses. Motor fitness is associated with the development of skilled movements, when the body gets used to a particular activity and becomes more adept at performing it through repeated practice. This is trained with the core stability work in Chapter 8.

Body composition is the amount of fat and lean body tissue (muscles, bones, organs and tissues) in the body. Whilst it does not relate to any particular type of activity it can be significantly affected by exercise. Regular exercise increases lean body weight (muscle) and decreases fat weight as muscle tissue burns more fat at rest and thus increases the metabolic rate. This is particularly relevant to postnatal weight loss.

Improving physical fitness

It is necessary to exercise to a level that places greater demands on the body in order to improve physical fitness. This is known as overload and results in physiological adaptations occurring in the body to cope with the new demands, often referred to as 'the training effect'. Progression must be slow and gradual to avoid doing too much too soon, and is dependent on the following factors:

• Previous fitness level
• Degree of fatigue
• Level of motivation
• Demands of the baby.

By altering the frequency, intensity, time and type of exercise, the body can be overloaded and fitness improved. These are known as the principles of training.

The principles of training

Frequency

It is important not to overdo it in the early weeks, particularly if any postnatal problems still persist or if sleep is interrupted. Despite the fact that exercise can often increase energy levels there is a risk of exhaustion if too much is attempted. From a practical point of view, it may be difficult to find the time to exercise on a regular basis, so if activities are incorporated into your daily routine, baby permitting, it will be much easier to be consistent. Cardiovascular exercise can be achieved through a long, brisk walk with the pushchair, and on returning home this could be followed by some of the essential floorwork exercises for muscular endurance and some stretching. Doing a little is often the best advice initially; 5–10 minutes every day building up to a full workout three times a week, depending on the time available. For exercise to be really effective it should be performed at a moderate intensity at least three times a week. More frequent sessions will have greater fitness benefits but exceeding five sessions may increase the risk of injury. Days off are essential to rest the body.

Intensity

The level at which exercise commences is most important. Previously fit women who continued to exercise during pregnancy may attempt to recommence at a similar level to that achieved prior to pregnancy. They may feel demoralised that the effects of pregnancy and delivery have taken a greater toll on the body than realised, but pushing themselves to uncomfortable levels will hinder full recovery and risk joint injury. Commencing at a gentle to moderate intensity allows time for the body to readjust and become familiar with the related skills of the activity. Intensity can be increased by changing the following four factors.

Resistance:
- gradient or incline used on a treadmill/bike;
- type of terrain when walking outdoors;
- positioning in relation to gravity and body weight;
- amount of resistance being lifted.

Repetitions:
- number of times the exercise is repeated.

Rate:
- pace of walking/jogging/cycling/stepping;
- speed of endurance exercises.*

Rest:
- length of time to rest between sets of repetitions;**
- length of active rest periods during cardiovascular training.

* The speed at which endurance exercises are performed is particularly important. Slow movements are much more demanding as they require the muscle to work over a longer period of time, but they are a much safer method. Faster movements often involve the assistance of momentum and carry the risk of joint overextension, which can be potentially damaging.

** Working in sets of repetitions is the most effective method of training for endurance. Resting the working muscle between sets allows a short period of recovery before repeating the exercise or lift, reducing the risk of early fatigue and providing a more effective challenge.

Time

A one-hour session is the optimum duration of a workout. This includes time for warming up and preparing the body, the workout itself (cardiovascular, muscular endurance or a combination of the two), and a period of cooling down and stretching. The duration of cardiovascular work should build gradually – 10 minutes may be sufficient to begin with, increasing to 20 or 30 minutes over an extended period of time. This does, of course, depend on the intensity of the activity as low-level exercise can be continued for longer. The relationship between duration and intensity should be carefully considered in all elements of the workout.

Type

The various types of exercise are discussed in the relevant chapters.

Exercise effectiveness

If physical fitness is to be improved, varying degrees of effort are essential.

- Cardiovascular exercise should induce a feeling of slight breathlessness, measured by the ability still to hold a conversation.
- Muscular endurance exercises should be of sufficient intensity to create an ache in the muscle being worked after about 12 repetitions. If more than 20 repetitions can be performed without any noticeable signs of work the resistance should be increased and the number of repetitions reduced.
- Stretches should be experienced as a feeling of mild tension in the muscle, which should be comfortable to hold for 6–8 seconds. Stretching should not be painful.

Training methods

Appropriate activities to train the components of physical fitness are comprehensively detailed in Chapters 8–11.

Summary

- Physical fitness encompasses cardiovascular fitness, muscular strength and endurance, flexibility and motor fitness. Programmes should aim to place demands on all these areas.
- To improve physical fitness the body must be overloaded. This is done by altering the frequency, intensity, time and type of exercise.
- Frequency should be increased gradually to the optimum three times a week. More than five sessions may increase the risk of injury.
- Intensity should be gentle to moderate to begin with and, depending on the frequency, may increase gradually over a period of time.
- Ten minutes of exercise may be all that circumstances allow, but this could increase to up to one hour depending on the intensity.
- Progression must be slow and gradual to avoid doing too much too soon.
- Overdoing it in the early weeks may be detrimental to your recovery.

PREPARING TO EXERCISE

How soon can formal exercise recommence?

It is recommended to wait until a satisfactory postnatal check-up has been completed; this generally occurs about six weeks after delivery. Whilst women who have had caesarean deliveries will have their check-up at the same time it is advisable for them to wait a further couple of weeks before commencing. This recovery period is essential to ensure that the uterus has retracted back into the pelvis, bleeding and discharge have ceased, and stitches have healed. It may take some time after the birth to feel ready for a formal exercise session, not only in terms of physical recovery but also to be sufficiently organised with the baby to make it out of the house in time for a deadline!

Can any exercises be undertaken before the postnatal check-up?

Women are usually given an exercise sheet on discharge from hospital, which include abdominal and pelvic floor strengthening to be performed at home, e.g. lying pelvic tilt, head and shoulder raises, static abdominal contractions and pelvic floor exercises. Although the importance of these exercises is emphasised and women are eager to commence, the demands of a new baby may prevent regular, or even occasional, undertaking. Incorporating exercise into the daily routine is the only way it can be regularly achieved:

- Postural exercises such as navel to spine and pelvic floor can be performed anywhere at any time but may be more convenient to remember when feeding or changing the baby.
- After nappy changing, while the baby is having a kick around on the floor.
- Before getting into bed or the bath, or even in the bath.
- Walking with the pushchair.

Gentle swimming may also be commenced before the check-up providing bleeding and discharge have completely finished.

Suitability for exercise

A postnatal check-up should ascertain whether there are any problems affecting suitability and participation in an exercise programme. The following areas are usually reviewed and discussed to varying degrees:

- retraction of the uterus back into the pelvis;
- cessation of red blood loss (other discharge may continue for longer);
- healing of perineum;
- perineum comfort;
- healing of caesarean scar;
- abdominal comfort following caesarean delivery;
- establishment of breastfeeding;
- condition of breasts;

- general physical condition;
- weight;
- blood pressure.

Occasionally the abdominal muscles may be checked for separation although this is not a routine test.

Preparing to exercise

Clothing

It is important to wear suitable clothing, appropriate to the chosen activity. Loose-fitting garments are preferred providing body alignment can still be seen. The breasts must be well supported by a bra designed to reduce movement; this will prevent overstretching of the ligaments and maintain comfort. Feeding bras do not provide sufficient support and although it may be practical to wear one if baby comes too it is recommended that a sports bra is worn over the top. Breast support in swimwear should also be considered, particularly if the activity is undertaken in shallow water.

Footwear

Appropriate footwear is essential for land-based cardiovascular and resistance activities. Specifically designed footwear is available for a variety of activities, and it is important to select the appropriate shoe for the intended activity which provides sufficient support and shock absorption.

Breastfeeding

Breastfeeding or expressing milk before exercising is recommended to reduce the weight of the breasts and the possibility of milk leaking. Plentiful amounts of fluid should be taken in before, during and after exercise to avoid dehydration, which is accentuated if breastfeeding.

Food intake

Exercise should not be undertaken on an empty stomach. It is recommended that a light carbohydrate snack is consumed approximately two to three hours before exercising to prevent a sudden drop in blood sugar with the onset of exercise. This is particularly relevant when breastfeeding.

Making time for exercise

This could be more difficult! A 'spare' two hours while baby sleeps in the morning is the ideal opportunity for exercise but there will probably be other jobs on the agenda! Routine domestic chores need to be undertaken, but if no help is available women must try to prioritise and complete only essential tasks. On the other hand, a disturbed night may necessitate sleep at this time. Exercise need not take up too much time; mini-programmes can be set to squeeze into a few minutes every day and extended programmes devised for those occasions when more time is available. Setting small, achievable goals is the only way forward and any additional accomplishments should be considered a bonus. Be aware that targets may not be reached every time!

And baby too . . .

There is, of course, no reason why some of the basic exercises should not be performed with the baby. Working out with the baby positioned next to mum can be a warm and fulfilling experience for both parties. Making eye contact, touching and talking to him will help to passify him for longer. Using the baby as a resistance should be avoided until mum's core strength has improved and baby has firm head control.

Tiredness or exhaustion

Exercise may be the last thing on a woman's mind when she is feeling tired and weary and longs for uninterrupted sleep. Gentle exercise can, however, be very therapeutic in re-energising and motivating. Whether it is a brisk walk with the pushchair or 10 minutes of essential floorwork, exercise should provide her with a welcome break from routine and an opportunity to re-focus on herself. However, previously fit women who have high expectations of themselves and have been used to pushing their bodies when they felt tired may have more difficulty recognising when the body is exhausted. In such cases the exercise session must make way for sleep.

Overdoing it

While exercise needs to be effective it should always be comfortable and achievable. By listening to her body a woman should be able to recognise when she is working effectively and when she is overdoing it.

- Effective exercise should feel comfortably hard. Slight discomfort and tiredness may be experienced and the muscles need to feel as if they are working but suffer no adverse after-effects.
- Overdoing it will result in aching muscles

and feeling excessively tired both immediately and/or on the following day.

Women need to learn to adjust their level of exercise accordingly and not battle on through the warning signs.

What are the warning signs?

Breathlessness, dizziness, and feelings of nausea are all signs that the body is being overstressed during cardiovascular exercise. Indications such as clumsiness, tripping and decreased co-ordination are not always recognised by the participant but will be noticed by an observant instructor. Uncomfortable burning sensations in the muscles during resistance work suggests the workload is too much and should be reduced. While these symptoms will generally occur during exercise, some may be experienced after exercise has finished or even the next day. Aching limbs and feelings of lethargy the next day are strong indicators that the body has been overworked.

When should exercise be stopped?

Pain of any sort is a warning sign which should never be ignored. Exercise should cease immediately or adaptations made to restore comfort. Never work through pain.

Summary

- Gentle exercises can be commenced at home in the first few weeks after the birth.
- A satisfactory postnatal check-up is necessary before commencing more vigorous exercise.
- Caesarean deliveries should wait 8–10 weeks.
- A good supporting bra should be worn to protect the breasts.
- Appropriate, supportive footwear should be worn where necessary.
- Milk should be expressed, or baby fed, before exercising.
- Increase fluid intake before, during and after exercise if breastfeeding.
- Eat 2–3 hours prior to exercising.
- Incorporate exercise into daily activities as much as possible.
- Exercise may need to be replaced with sleep on some occasions.
- The level of exercise must be comfortable and achievable.
- Women should learn to recognise when they have had enough.
- Exercise should stop immediately, and adaptations made, if pain is experienced.

CORE STABILITY TRAINING

What is core stability?

Also known as spinal stability, this term relates to the ability of the body to maintain control and balance during movement. It is governed by stabilising muscles which lie deep within the body's musculature, so their movements cannot be obviously observed, but their role is to provide support for the larger actions of the body.

Which are the core muscles?

Four muscles lying deep inside the trunk – transversus abdominis, multifidus, diaphragm and pelvic floor – and their interconnective tissue are considered the key stabilisers.

Multifidus, a deep spinal muscle, is enveloped in the thoracolumbar fascia from which transversus abdominis originates. The diaphragm interdigitates with transversus abdominis in its attachment and the pelvic floor is on the same neural loop as TrA.

Activation of TrA tenses the thoracolumbar fascia and co-activates the diaphragm and pelvic floor muscles to form an enclosed abdominal ring – termed 'a cylinder of stability' by Hodges (1999). This generates increased intra-abdominal pressure which increases lumbar stability.

Why are they so important?

Key postural muscles are often weak and unable to provide support to functional movements. If the deep muscular system does

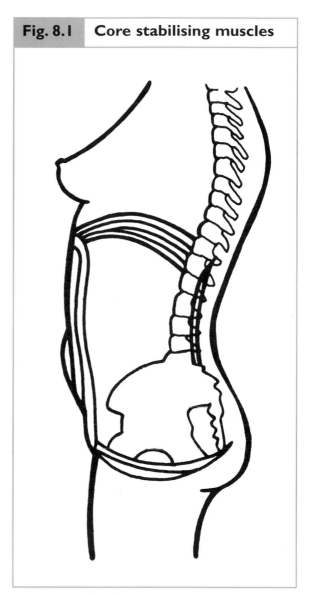

Fig. 8.1   Core stabilising muscles

not engage, the larger superficial muscles will be activated to take over the work. These larger muscles are designed for dynamic movement and are not intended to work for prolonged periods of time. Their overuse causes muscular tension as they remain permanently contracted, and results in postural changes and pain! Unfortunately conventional exercises do not address these muscles as they focus predominantly on the more visible mobilising system to improve strength and definition.

How do the core muscles work?

These slow-twitch muscles function at very low intensities (20–30% of maximum voluntary contraction), and are slow to fatigue. Required to sustain the workload, their recruitment will fluctuate in intensity depending on the degree of force exerted by the limbs. Once activated, they will engage more easily in the future, but they need to be stimulated 30,000 times for this response to be autonomic. Unfortunately this information is not transferable between movements, which necessitates the programming of their activation into all movement patterns commonly used.

Benefits of postnatal core training

- Targets the key areas of weakness.
- Teaches the body to switch off dominant muscles.
- Releases muscular tension in unwanted areas.
- Replicates functional movements needed for everyday life.
- Challenges the whole body as an integrated unit by increasing co-ordination and proprioception.
- Develops freedom and ease of movement – if an exercise looks easy the stabilising system is probably working.

All the TrA exercises on pages 16–26 in Chapter 2 are for core stability.

The Foam Roller

Introduction to the foam roller

The roller is an excellent tool for learning to control the spine via the deep stabilising muscles. It helps the body to switch off muscles that don't need to work, and recruit a low-level response from the muscles that need to stabilise, while allowing freedom of movement. It is also fun to use!

It can be used to lie on, supine or prone, to sit on or to place under or on top of the body. Lying supine on the roller massages the spine, increases circulation and stimulates the discs to absorb fluid. All positions encourage neutral spinal alignment. Pregnancy postural changes can be addressed as the roller helps to identify areas of tightness, weakness and restriction. Prone positions may need adapting for breast comfort.

The following exercises are intended to explore the basic concepts of the roller and introduce the idea to instructors. It is a complex tool to teach but has enormous potential; further training is strongly recommended through Stability in Action (*see* Useful Contacts for further details).

Supine exercises

Getting on

Whether the roller is butted against the wall or freestanding, the transition to supine lying is the same and should be regarded as an exercise in itself.

Ex 8.1	**Getting Down**

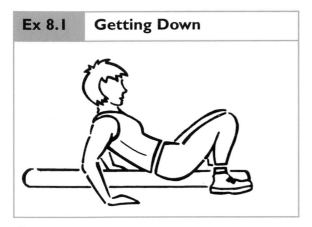

Preparation

Butt one end of the roller against the wall and take a wide stance astride it as close to the wall as you can. Keeping the legs turned out, away from the wall, draw navel to spine and sit down. If you are freestanding, clip the ankle bones either side of the roller and bend with knees aligned in parallel. Lean gently back and place your hands on the floor.*

Action

Draw navel to spine to pelvic tilt and slowly roll down through the spine until you are lying flat. It may be necessary to tighten the gluteals gently to feel the lumbar spine curling down. Keep the abdominals held in throughout and try to feel each of the vertebrae pressing into the roller as you move down. Aim to get the spine as straight as possible on the surface of the roller and make a mental note of areas that appear to deviate. Draw navel to spine and lift, one leg at a time, to the wall and place hip-width apart with a 90-degree angle at knees and hips. Find your neutral alignment, then rest arms on the floor with palms rotated upwards. Relax and sink into the roller, breathing naturally.

Technique tips

• This might feel quite uncomfortable initially so it is important to allow a few minutes for your body to settle into the roller.
• It is likely your back will tighten to resist the pressure created by the dense surface of the roller, so it may take some time for the muscles to relax.
• Put equal weight on both feet.
• Keep pelvis level.
• Keep chest wide and ribcage in contact with the roller.
• Align head – eye-line to ceiling.
• If discomfort is still felt after a few minutes, particularly in the thoracic spine, it may be necessary to put a thin cushion or thick towel on top of the roller.
• Sacral/coccyx discomfort could be helped by placing a thin sponge underneath the area to reduce pressure.

*Cautions: Great care should be taken to avoid doming of the abdominals during this transition. Exercising at the wall may be unsuitable for women suffering from SPD as the transition into position may stress the joint.

Melt down

Remain in the above position for up to five minutes. The longer you remain in this position the more you will be able to release unwanted

Ex 8.2	**Melt Down**

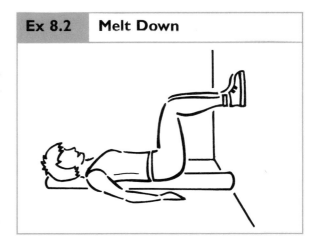

tension. Feel your body slowly giving in to the pressure of the roller and allowing the muscles to release. The vertebra should begin to open and the chest widen as the body melts and becomes one with the support. This is extremely valuable in itself – if you only have time to do this, it will be time well spent.

Getting off

Moving off the roller may feel a little uncomfortable, particularly if you have spent some time on it. Draw navel to spine and roll the whole body over to the side, as one unit and push the roller out of the way. Lie back on the floor and enjoy the 'softness' of the new surface. Experience the openness created in the chest and the increased length of the spine. Stay there for a few minutes and relax.

The following exercises from Chapter 2 can be transposed to the roller on or off the wall.

Before commencing, try to straighten the spine on the roller and adopt neutral spinal alignment.

Shoulder release

Purpose: to release muscular tension and induce freedom of movement.

Preparation

As above at the wall, in neutral spinal alignment. Both arms lifted to the ceiling at shoulder level. Shoulders relaxed.

Action

Imagine your arms are suspended from the ceiling so the shoulders can just relax. Inhale and float both arms up to the ceiling feeling the shoulder-blades lifting around your side. Exhale, drawing navel to spine and release the shoulder-blades down to the roller, keeping the elbows straight.

Technique tips

- Imagine your arms are suspended from the ceiling.
- Let go in the shoulder.
- Keep open in the collar bone.
- Feel the shoulder-blades relaxing around the roller as you lower.
- Maintain neutral alignment throughout.
- Avoid pressing the feet into the wall.

Scissor arms

(*See* page 19)

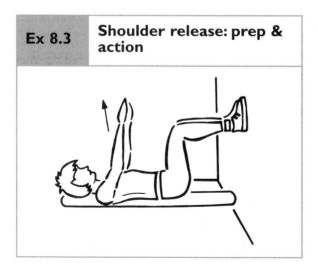

Ex 8.3	Shoulder release: prep & action

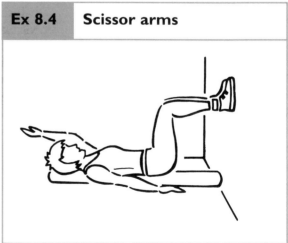

Ex 8.4	Scissor arms

Chest flye

(as page 19)

This is particularly beneficial on the roller as it helps to lengthen tight pectoral muscles which frequently shorten with breastfeeding. Pause with the arms open to the side to allow the muscles to relax and lengthen. This position may induce a nerve stretch, with tingling in the shoulder, down the inside of the arm into the fingers. If this becomes uncomfortable, avoid pausing in position, keep the movement continuous but slow.

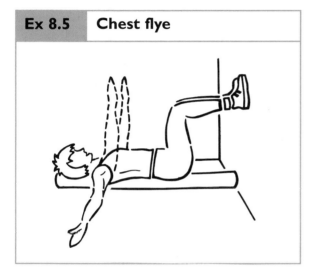

| Ex 8.5 | Chest flye |

Arm circle

(*See* page 20)

Pelvic tilt

(*See* page 30)

Knee raise

(*See* page 21)

Heel and elbow raise

Purpose: to use TrA to stabilise the spine whilst the arms and legs move.

Preparation

As before, with elbows bent, resting on the floor and fingertips on hip bones.

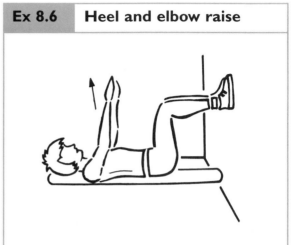

| Ex 8.6 | Heel and elbow raise |

Action

Inhale, and as you exhale draw navel to spine and lift one heel off the wall, at the same time lifting the opposite elbow off the floor. Inhale to lower and transfer weight onto the other side. Repeat on alternate sides.

Technique tips

- Check the alignment of the pelvis with the fingertips – avoid rocking from side to side.
- Maintain neutral spinal alignment.
- Avoid pushing into the wall.
- Perform slowly with control.

Progression

Lift both elbows off floor and continue with alternate heel raises.

Wall walking

Purpose: to use TrA to stabilise the spine whilst transferring body weight from side to side.

Preparation
As above with elbows bent, lifted off the floor, fingertips on hip bones.

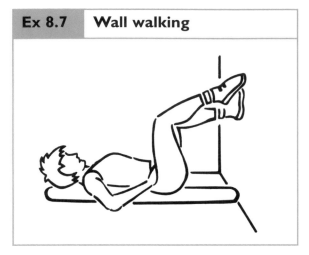

Ex 8.7	**Wall walking**

Action
Inhale, and as you exhale draw navel to spine and hinge at the toe joints, lifting the arches of the feet as high as possible. Progress by peeling the whole foot off the wall and walk on the spot.

Technique tips
- Maintain neutral alignment.
- Avoid rocking the pelvis from side to side.
- Avoid pushing into the wall on the supporting side.
- Try to keep the elbows off the floor if possible.

Supine lying in the centre

Leg slide

(*See* page 18)

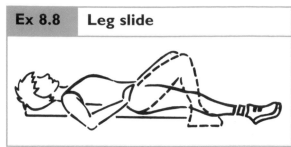

Ex 8.8	**Leg slide**

Pelvic tilt

(*See* page 30)

Bridge

(*See* page 30)
NB Range must be reduced on the roller.

All arm exercises

(*See* pages 19–20)

Leg slide with arm combination

(*See* pages 19–20)

Knee raise

(*See* page 21)

Toe touch

(*See* page 23)
NB Range must be reduced on the roller.

Thoracic extension

Purpose: to mobilise thoracic spine and improve kyphotic posture.

Preparation
Lie supine with knees bent up, feet flat. Place the roller lengthways under the lower border of

the shoulder-blades and lean on it. Use both hands to support the head firmly in neutral, with elbows facing forwards. Tilt the pelvis to prevent the lower back hyperextending.

Ex 8.9	**Thoracic extension**

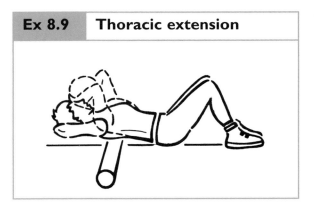

Action
Inhale to prepare, and as you exhale draw navel to spine and gently extend the upper spine over the roller, opening the elbows to the side. Allow the head to move with you but maintain it in neutral alignment. Draw down in the ribcage to prevent overextension. Pause to inhale and maintain control, exhale to draw navel to spine and curl the body back up.

Technique tips
• Maintain pelvic tilt to avoid hyperextending lumbar spine.
• Draw the shoulder-blades down to release the ribcage.
• Maintain neutral cervical alignment.
• Bring the arms further forward if this pulls in the shoulder.
• Avoid leading with the head on recovery.

Caution: This is a complex exercise to perform correctly and needs careful observation

Single leg stretch
(*See* page 24)

Ex 8.10	**Single leg stretch**

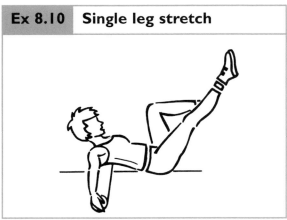

Lying supine with roller placed lengthways under shoulder blades, arm outstretched holding roller. The roller is a useful aid to spinal flexion in this exercise and is extremely effective in exercising TrA and RA. Pelvic tilting is recommended to prevent lumbar hyperextension.

Prone exercises

Scapular stabilisation

Purpose: to increase shoulder-blade stabilisation and improve upper body posture.

Preparation
Lie prone with legs together and arms reaching above the head in an open V. Position the roller firmly underneath the palms and draw your shoulder blades down your back. Lift your elbows off the floor and relax the forehead to the floor or on a small cushion.

Ex 8.11	**Scapular stabilisation**

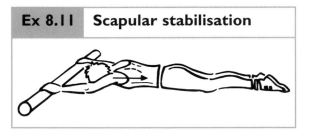

Action

Inhale to prepare, and as you exhale draw navel to spine and slowly draw the roller downwards, keeping the elbows straight so that the shoulder-blades move further down your back. This will be a small movement. Inhale to release and return the arms to the extended position, keeping the shoulders relaxed.

Technique tips
• Extend your legs out from the hips.
• Keep the wrists lifted.
• Draw ribs to hips throughout.
• Keep the abdominals lightly held in.
• If the back feels uncomfortable, place a small cushion underneath the abdomen.

NB Pressure on the breasts may be relieved by rolling a towel up between the breasts and placing pillows above and below the chest. This exercise may have to be postponed until the breasts feel more comfortable in the prone position.

Scapular stabilisation with thoracic extension

Draw the roller downwards as above and continue the movement by lifting the upper body to extend the thoracic spine. Maintain connection between rib and hips and keep the movement only in thoracic spine. Whilst some extension will occur in lumbar spine, it should

Ex 8.12	**Scapular stabilisation**

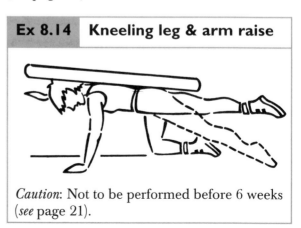

not be allowed to hyperextend. This is an excellent exercise to improve kyphotic posture.

Kneeling abdominal raise
(*See* page 22)

Ex 8.13	**Kneeling abdominal raise**

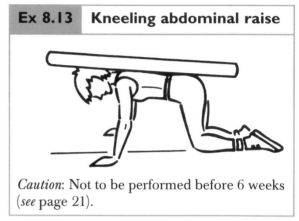

Caution: Not to be performed before 6 weeks (*see* page 21).

Place the roller along the spine to check neutral alignment. Points of contact should be sacrum, lower ribs and back of head. Perform the abdominal raise without changing spinal alignment, and keeping the roller balanced along the spine.

Kneeling leg & arm raise
(*See* page 22)

Ex 8.14	**Kneeling leg & arm raise**

Caution: Not to be performed before 6 weeks (*see* page 21).

With roller balanced along the spine as above. Build up to the complete exercise with the following stages:

- Arm lift
- Leg slide foot on floor
- Arm lift and leg slide together
- Leg lift
- Arm lift and leg lift together

Stretches

Seated hamstring stretch

As page 116 with roller placed lengthways under heel, hands on the floor behind, and back lifted. Push down on hands and move your sit bones back, allowing the roller to move with you. Take care not to allow the knees to hyperextend. After stretching, sit on the roller with hands on the floor either side, and move it backwards and forwards underneath the hamstrings. This gives a great massage for tight muscles!

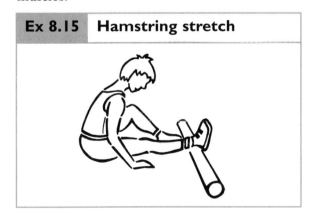

Ex 8.15	Hamstring stretch

Seated gluteal stretch

(as page 116) Sit lengthways on the roller. After stretching, allow the roller to move backwards and forwards underneath the buttock to massage the muscle.

Pectoral stretch

Purpose: to lengthen pectoralis minor and increase mobility in the shoulder.

Preparation
Lie supine on the roller, with neutral spinal alignment. Reach the arms out to the side at shoulder height with elbows bent to 90 degrees, forearms vertical to the ceiling.

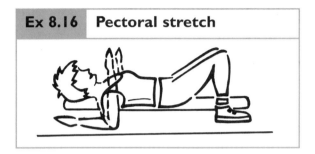

Ex 8.16	Pectoral stretch

Action
Inhale, and as you exhale draw navel to spine and move the forearm slowly backwards towards the floor, keeping the wrist and forearm aligned. Keep the elbows off the floor. Hold the position at its farthest point, continuing to breathe, and try to relax.

Technique tips
- Maintain neutral spinal alignment.
- Do not allow the ribcage to lift.
- Allow the arms to relax – avoid hanging on.
- Aim to get the wrist to the floor.
- Keep the elbow lifted.

The Ball

Introduction to the ball

The ball is incredibly effective in building functional strength as it challenges the whole body to react as an integrated unit rather than working isolated muscle groups.

Exercising on an unstable base requires balance and this necessitates the recruitment of many deep stabilising muscles to maintain it. Since most of these muscles are generally underused, exercising on the ball will increase core strength and improve posture. No matter which body part is being worked on the ball, the core will always be trained, even during stretches. It is an excellent method of muscular rehabilitation for postnatal women.

The following is a small selection of suitable postnatal exercises on the ball. Further training on the ball is recommended for the inexperienced instructor.

Seated posture

Purpose: to redress posture in sitting.

Preparation
Ensure the ball is the correct size for you and inflated sufficiently. Incorrect size will cause misalignment of the knees and hips which may incur injury. The feet should be hip-width apart, flat on the floor, with a 90-degree angle at the hips and the knees. Hands should be resting on thighs or the ball.

Ex 8.17	Seated posture

- Position yourself directly on your sit bones.
- Maintain neutral spinal alignment.
- Lengthen the spine away from your sit bones.
- Slide the shoulder-blades down.

NB You may need to begin with feet a little wider than hip-width to help you balance. Narrowing the width of your base will reduce stability and make the exercises more challenging.

Sitting tall on the ball aligns the body naturally and safely and places the least strain on the body. Slumping increases the ball's instability. Sit for a few minutes, breathing naturally, maintaining correct body alignment. Unassisted sitting is an endurance activity, so don't overdo it.

Seated exercises

Seated pelvic tilt

Purpose: to shorten RA and use TrA to stabilise in a balanced position.

Preparation
Start seated as above, hand on thighs or the ball.

Action
Inhale to prepare, and as you exhale draw navel to spine and tilt the pelvis. Use the abdominals rather than the buttocks to lift the pubic bone and curve the lumbar spine, rolling the ball underneath you. Release and return to neutral sitting, rolling the ball back.

Seated hip circle

Purpose: to mobilise the lower back.

Preparation
Start seated as above.

Action

Move through the pelvic tilt and continue the hips around in a circle. Make the movement as large as possible but avoid slumping into an anterior tilt. Return to the upright seated position and lift away from the sit bones.

Seated heel raise

Purpose: to mobilise the feet and use TrA to stabilise the spine.

Preparation
Start seated as above.

Action
Inhale to prepare and as you exhale draw navel to spine and lift the heels, rolling the ball forward. Inhale to roll back.

Technique tips
- Maintain neutral alignment throughout.
- Aim to lift the arches of the feet as high as possible with weight travelling through the centre of each foot and equally distributed across the toe joints.
- To progress this into an effective strengthening exercise for the calves, lean the upper body forward and rest hands or elbows on thighs.

Seated knee raise

Purpose: to use TrA to stabilise and control lower body movements.

Preparation
Seated as above.

Action
Inhale to prepare, and as you exhale draw navel to spine and transfer your weight onto the left foot, before floating the right leg off the

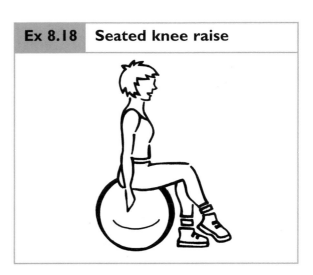

Ex 8.18   Seated knee raise

floor and lifting the knee up to hip height. Inhale to lower and transfer weight onto the other foot.

Technique tips
- Maintain neutral spine and lift away from sit bones.
- Avoid pushing down onto the other foot.
- Perform slowly to encourage the stabilising muscles to work for longer.
- Maintain correct seated posture throughout.

Seated scissor arms

Purpose: to use TrA to stabilise and control upper body movements.

Preparation
Seated as above in neutral spinal alignment with arms resting on thighs.

Action
Inhale and lift both arms up in front of chest, keeping shoulders relaxed. As you exhale draw navel to spine and scissor one arm up above the head and the other down by your side. Inhale to return both arms to chest height and exhale to change. Repeat 8 times on each side.

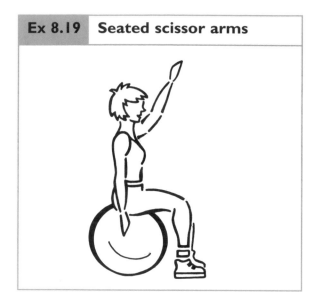

Ex 8.19	Seated scissor arms

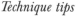

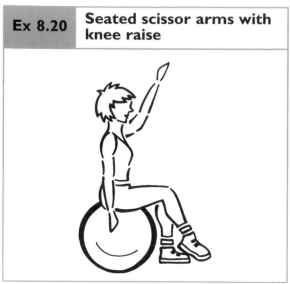

Ex 8.20	Seated scissor arms with knee raise

Technique tips
- Maintain neutral spinal alignment as the arm lifts.
- Keep the ribcage drawn down.
- Lengthen both arms as far away from the shoulders as possible.
- Slide the shoulder-blades down your back throughout.
- Lift away from your sit bones.
- Keep the movement slow and controlled.

Seated scissor arms with knee raise

Purpose: to use TrA to stabilise and control co-ordinated movements.

Preparation
Seated as above in neutral spinal alignment with hands resting on thighs.

Action
Inhale and float both arms in front of the chest, keeping the shoulders sliding down. As you exhale, draw navel to spine and lift the right

knee up in front and scissor the arms with left up and right arm down. Inhale to lower the foot to the floor and return the arms to chest height. Exhale to repeat on the other side.

Technique tips
- Maintain neutral spine throughout.
- Avoid pressing down into the supporting foot.
- Peel the foot off the floor and float the knee up.
- Keep the ribcage and shoulder-blades drawn down.
- Lengthen both arms as far away from the shoulders as possible.
- Keep the transition smooth.
- Lift away from your sit bones.
- Keep the movement slow and controlled.

Supine exercises

Supine roll down

Purpose: to use RA to lower the body and TrA to stabilise the spine. This can be used as warm-up to increase body awareness on the ball and is

Ex 8.21 Supine roll down

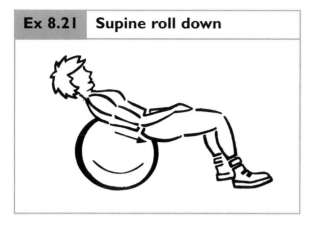

a transition to the supine position for further exercises.

Preparation
Seated as above in neutral spinal alignment with hands resting on the ball.

Action
Inhale to prepare, and as you exhale draw navel to spine, perform pelvic tilt and walk the feet forward. Allow the ball to roll up your back until it fits snugly into the lumbar vertebrae. Release the pelvic tilt and allow the spine to fall into neutral. Pause in this position for a few seconds, keeping the head aligned with the spine. Draw navel to spine and roll back up to seated, keeping the spine in contact with the ball throughout. Use your arms on the ball to help you roll up. Repeat slowly several times.

Technique tips
• Knees should be flexed to 90 degrees in the supine position.
• Ensure the abdomen remains flat by maintaining navel to spine.
• Maintain correct cervical alignment.
• Support with one hand behind the head if tension increases in the neck and shoulders.
• Make the movements up and down smooth and continuous.

• Wider foot base will aid balance and stabilisation.

Caution: If the abdominals begin to dome, return to the seated position and repeat, ensuring you have drawn navel to spine. If doming continues postpone this exercise until strength has been regained in TrA.

Progression
When you feel more confident, rest your hands on your thighs as you roll down, or lift them in front at chest height.

Supine pelvic tilt

Purpose: to shorten RA and use TrA to stabilise and control the balanced position.

Preparation
Perform the supine roll down as above and pause in position with hands resting on thighs.

Action
Inhale to prepare, and as you exhale draw navel to spine and lift the pubic bone up towards breastbone. Inhale to release and return to neutral spinal alignment. Perform several times or roll back up to seated position and perform the whole sequence.

Ex 8.22 Supine pelvic tilt

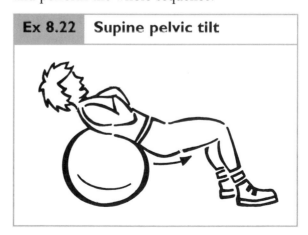

Technique tips
- Use the abdominals, not the gluteals, to create the movement.
- Draw hips to ribs but keep the ribcage down into the ball.
- Keep the upper body relaxed throughout.
- If discomfort is experienced in the neck and shoulders place both hands behind the head.
- Perform with feet together to decrease stabilisation and increase the challenge.

Supine curl-up

Purpose: to strengthen RA in a balanced position and use TrA to stabilise the spine. Performed on the ball, RA is able to work through a greater range of movement.

Caution: This is a Level 3 abdominal exercise (*see* page 34) and should not be attempted until Levels 1 and 2 can be competently performed.

Preparation
As above – supine roll down position with the lumbar spine into the ball. Place both hands behind the head for support and lengthen through the back of the neck.

Ex 8.23	Supine curl-up

Action
Inhale to prepare, and as you exhale draw navel to spine, sliding ribs to hips as you curl the upper body forward. Do not allow the pelvis to tilt. Inhale to hold, keeping the abdomen held in flat, exhale to lower slowly to start position, keeping navel drawn into spine.

Technique tips
- Keep feet hip-width apart.
- Slide ribs to hips as you curl the trunk.
- Keep the abdominals held in flat throughout.
- Feel the back in contact with the ball at all times.
- Maintain neutral spinal alignment – do not pelvic tilt.
- Slide the shoulder-blades down your back.
- Keep the head and neck supported throughout.
- Maintain correct cervical alignment.
- If doming occurs, stop immediately and check technique.

NB Placing both hands behind the head increases the intensity of the exercise but may be necessary to reduce neck strain. It may be preferable to use just one hand, providing this does not alter balance and stability.

Pectoral stretch

Purpose: to lengthen tight pectorals incurred by postural changes of pregnancy and breastfeeding.

Preparation
Supine roll down.

Action
Lay your head back to rest on the ball and release into it. Draw navel to spine as you take your arms out to the side just above shoulder height and lengthen the arms away from the shoulder. Hold for a few seconds, releasing into the ball.

Ex 8.24	Pectoral stretch

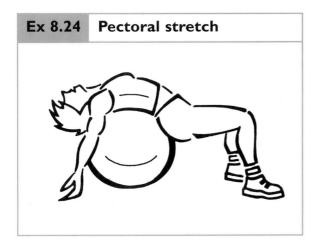

Ex 8.25	Kneeling abdominal raise with arm lift

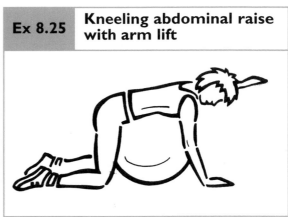

Technique tips
- Allow the hips to drop to keep the lower back into the ball.
- Feel a strong stretch across the front of the shoulder and into the chest.
- This feeling may radiate down the inside of the arm and into the fingers.
- Keep the head supported on the ball.

Alternative
If this causes uncomfortable tingling down the inside of the arm and into the fingers, avoid holding the position and perform as a slow, continuous movement.

Prone exercises

Caution: The exercises in this section are not suitable until after six weeks. *See* page 21.

Kneeling abdominal raise
Purpose: to strengthen TrA.

Preparation
Kneeling over the ball with equal weight on hands and knees. Relax the abdomen into the ball. If this position is uncomfortable for your

breasts, deflate the ball a little or go on to the next exercise.

Action
Inhale, and as you exhale draw navel to spine and lift abdomen away from the ball. Inhale to release the abdomen into the ball.

Technique tips
- Keep the head aligned with spine.
- Keep buttocks relaxed and hips on the ball.
- Use the abdominals to create the movement.

Progression
Repeat as above with one hand lifting off the floor and extending above the head at shoulder height as you exhale. Keep the head aligned, do not allow it to hyperextend. See next exercise for technique tips.

Abdominal raise with arm lift
Purpose: to strengthen lower trapezius to improve upper body posture and use TrA to stabilise spine.

Preparation
Lie over the ball with hands and feet on floor, equal weight distributed between the four

points. This position (prone balance) may be more comfortable for the breasts than the previous exercise.

Ex 8.26 | Prone balance position

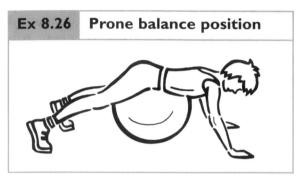

Action

Inhale to prepare, and as you exhale draw navel to spine and lift one hand off the floor extending the arm above the head at shoulder height. Keep the head aligned, do not allow it to hyperextend. Inhale to lower and release into the ball.

Technique tips
- Lift the abdomen away from the ball.
- Lengthen your fingers away from the shoulder.
- Draw the shoulder blades down.
- Keep navel to spine as you extend the arm away.
- Maintain neutral alignment throughout.

Abdominal raise with leg lift

Purpose: to strengthen gluteus maximus to improve posture and use TrA to stabilise torso.

Preparation
Prone balance position as above.

Action
Inhale to prepare, and as you exhale draw navel to spine and lift one foot off the floor, extending the leg away. Inhale to lower.

Ex 8.27 | Abdominal raise with leg lift

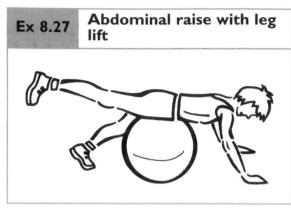

Technique tips
- Feet hip-width apart.
- Hands shoulder-width apart.
- Keep shoulder-blades sliding down.
- Keep the hip on the ball.
- Extend the leg away from the hip as you lift.
- Lift the abdomen away from the ball with each lift.
- Maintain neutral spinal alignment throughout.
- Alternating legs increases the stabilisation challenge.

Swimming

Purpose: to use TrA to stabilise the spine as the gluteus maximus and lower trapezius work to improve posture. This is a combination of the two exercises above, i.e. abdominal raise with arm and opposite leg lift.

Ex 8.28 | Swimming

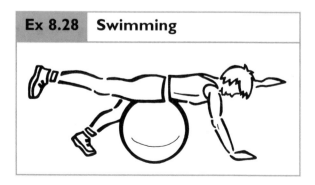

Preparation
As above, with hands and feet opened wider to the side for added stability.

Action
Inhale to prepare, and as you exhale draw navel to spine lifting right arm and left leg off the floor. Inhale to lower, exhale to repeat on the other side.

Technique tips
• Draw the abdomen away from the ball.
• Feel a diagonal reach from fingers through to opposite toes.
• Draw shoulder blades down.
• Maintain neutral spine (particularly watch lumbar and cervical).
• Keep the head aligned.
• Lift through the ribcage to maintain correct alignment.
• Keep the transition smooth and controlled.

Progression
Narrow the base by bringing feet in to hip-width apart and hands to shoulder-width apart. This reduces stability and makes the exercise more challenging.

Back stretch

Purpose: to stretch tight spinal extensors, reduce spinal compression and relax!

NB Do not attempt this stretch with a full stomach or full breasts!

Preparation
Kneel over the ball with hands and knees on the floor.

Action
Roll gently forward over the ball until your knees are lifted and your elbows bent.

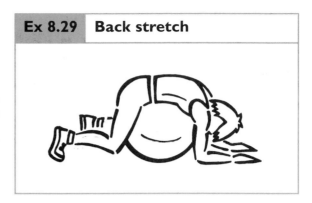

| Ex 8.29 | **Back stretch** |

Relax your head and knees towards the floor and allow the weight from both ends to stretch the spine around the ball. Hold for a few seconds and focus the breath into the back of the ribcage. Feel the spine releasing further.

Technique tips
• Curl the spine around the ball as much as possible.
• Let go and relax.
• Allow gravity to lengthen the spine from both ends.
• Long hair should be tied back, as it may get caught under the ball as you roll forward!

NB If the breasts feel uncomfortable, release some air from the ball. Alternatively, kneel and hug the ball in front of you. Relax your head to one side.

Back extension

Purpose: to strengthen lumbar extensors and use TrA to stabilise spine.

Preparation
Lie over the ball in the prone balance position as before. Move the weight back onto your feet, turning your toes in and heels out. Place your hands on the lower part of the ball and relax forward over it.

Ex 8.30	**Back extension**

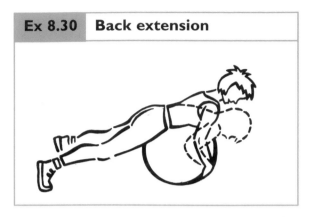

Action

Inhale, and as you exhale draw navel to spine and extend the spine up and back, lifting the upper body away from the ball. Avoid pushing with the hands. Inhale to lower, keeping the abdominals lifted to maintain control.

Technique tips
- Keep the head aligned throughout (placing a small ball under the chin will help to maintain neutral cervical alignment).
- Maintain navel to spine to support the back during both phases of the movement.
- Concentrate on drawing the shoulder-blades down as you lift, avoid squeezing them together.
- Lift the abdomen away from the ball.
- Lengthen your torso away from your feet.
- Keep your buttocks relaxed.
- Keep the movement small to begin with and progress to a larger range as strength increases.

Progression

Place hands on the back of the thighs and reach down the leg as you extend. Maintain neutral alignment throughout. The higher you are able to lift the greater the likelihood of the head dropping back, so watch out for cervical alignment.

Prone flye

Purpose: to strengthen mid-trapezius to assist with correction of pregnancy posture and use TrA to stabilise spine.

Preparation

Begin in prone balance position as before with feet apart. Move the weight back onto your feet, so your breasts are comfortable, and place your hands on the lower part of the ball. Keep the upper body lifted.

Ex 8.31	**Prone flye**

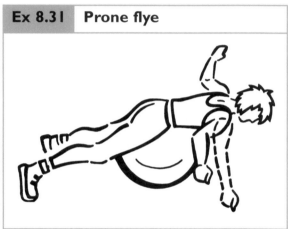

Action

Inhale, and as you exhale draw navel to spine as you slide the shoulder-blades down and back and lift the arms up to the side. Keep the elbows bent and lift from the back of the arm. Inhale to lower and repeat.

Technique tips
- Draw shoulder-blades down your back as you lift the arms.
- Maintain navel to spine throughout.
- Keep the head aligned with the rest.
- Keep the lower ribcage into the ball.
- Lift the abdomen away from the ball.
- Open the arms wide and full.
- Lead with the back of the arm.

Progression
Straighten the arms out to the side.

Press-ups

Purpose: to strengthen pectorals and triceps and use TrA to stabilise spine.

Preparation
From the prone balance position with legs together, walk the hands forward so the legs are lifted parallel to the floor and the ball is centred under the hips. Hands wider than shoulders with fingers facing forward, arms straight. Draw the shoulder-blades down and lengthen the spine.

Ex 8.32	Press-ups

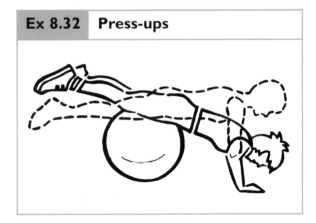

Action
Inhale to prepare and as you exhale draw navel to spine and lengthen the back. Inhale to bend the elbows and lower the upper body towards the floor, keeping the head aligned with the spine. Exhale to extend the elbows and return to starting position.

Technique tips
• Maintain navel to spine.
• Keep the head aligned with the spine.
• Check elbows over wrists as you bend.
• Avoid flexing the elbows below 90 degrees.

• Avoid locking out the elbows as they extend.
• Keep the shoulder-blades sliding down your back.

Caution: If the abdominals are weak, the spine will sag and neutral alignment will be lost. In such cases this exercise should be postponed until TrA strength has been gained.

Progression
Walk the hands further forward so the ball rolls onto the thighs, increasing stabilisation and length of lever.

Standing exercise

Standing squats

Purpose: to strengthen gluteus maximus, hamstrings and quadriceps to improve posture and use TrA to stabilise the spine.

Preparation
Standing at the wall, with the ball positioned between the lower back and the wall. Walk the feet out one or two paces and stand hip-width apart. Place hands on hips and lean back onto the ball.

Ex 8.33	Standing squats

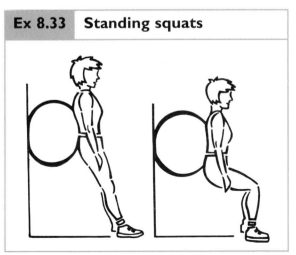

Action

Inhale to prepare and as you exhale, draw navel to spine and bend the knees so the ball rolls up your back. Inhale to straighten the knees and return to starting position. Ensure knees are over ankles as you bend – if not, walk the feet further forward before continuing

Technique tips
- Maintain navel to spine throughout.
- Avoid flexing the knees below 90 degrees.
- Maintain knees in parallel.
- Keep the upper body lifted in neutral alignment.
- Press down through the heels to straighten up.
- Lean into the ball.

Progression

Increase the length of hold in the squat, maintaining alignment as above.

Summary

- Core stability is the ability of the body to maintain control and balance during movement.
- It is governed by the deep stabilising muscles – transversus abdominis, multifidus, diaphragm and pelvic floor.
- These postural muscles are required to work at a low intensity for long periods.
- Postural muscles are often weak.
- Larger, dynamic muscles often take over the stabilising role.
- Overuse of the superficial muscles increases muscular tension and imbalance.
- Core stability training teaches the body to switch off dominant muscles.
- Core muscles need to be stimulated 30,000 times for the response to be autonomic.
- Information is not transferable between movements.
- Activation needs to be programmed into all movement patterns.
- Core stability training challenges the whole body as one integrated unit.
- It replicates functional movement and develops freedom and ease of movement.
- Conventional exercises do not address these muscles.

SELECTED POSTNATAL EXERCISES

How to use this programme

The following exercises can be performed immediately following the birth and should be encouraged frequently throughout the day.

- Navel to spine contractions in any position except 4 point kneeling (*see* page 21)
- Pelvic floor exercises in any position except 4 point kneeling (*see* page 42)

Some of the exercises described in the warm-up (*see* page 90) could be included as well. From about day eight, depending on how she is feeling, a woman can introduce some of the other exercises for TrA in a variety of positions. Progressions are indicated for many exercises, but avoid moving to the next exercise until the recommended level has been achieved and maintained. TrA exercises should feature very strongly in any programme.

Correct posture and alignment should be demonstrated throughout the programme.

Correct posture

- Stand with the feet hip-width apart.
- Distribute weight evenly between both feet.
- Transmit weight evenly between big toe, little toe and heel.
- Soften the knees and align them over the ankles.
- Find your neutral spine (*see* page 6).
- Draw navel to spine.
- Lengthen the spine.
- Slide the shoulders down and open the chest.

- Lengthen the neck, keeping the chin parallel to the floor.
- Look straight ahead.

Fig 9.1	**Correct posture**

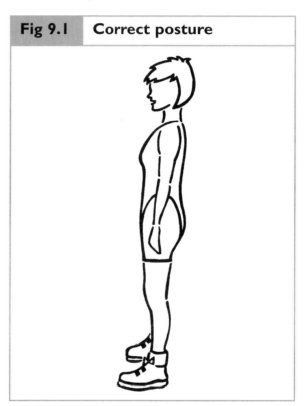

Warm-up

Mobility/pulse-raising movements.

Marching on the spot

Purpose: to warm the muscles and increase circulation.

89

Preparation
Stand tall with good posture, neutral spine, arms relaxed by sides.

Ex 9.1	**Marching on the spot**

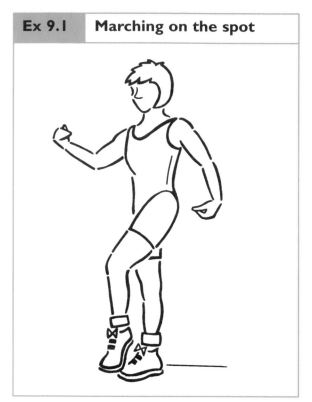

Action
March briskly on the spot, raising the knees to a comfortable height in front. Bend the elbows and move the arms forwards and back with each step. Maintain navel to spine and lifted chest. Continue until body begins to feel warmer. Repeat again before stretching.

Technique tips
- Think of the action as lifting the knees up rather than putting the feet down – this reduces stress on the joints.
- Avoid rocking the hips from side to side.
- Keep the knees aligned – avoid rolling them in.

Shoulder circle

Purpose: to mobilise the shoulder joint.

Preparation
Stand tall with good posture, neutral spine, arms relaxed by sides.

Ex 9.2	**Shoulder circle**

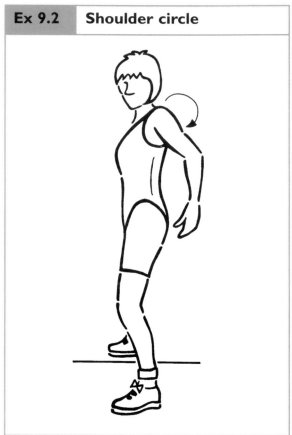

Action
Slowly circle one shoulder forwards, up, back and down in a large exaggerated way. Maintain navel to spine and lifted chest. Perform with the desired number of repetitions before changing sides.

Technique tips
- Emphasise the backward and downward

movements.
- Keep both hips facing forward.
- Maintain upright stance.
- Keep the knees soft.
- Keep the movement slow and controlled.

Side bend

Purpose: to mobilise the spine.

Preparation
Stand tall with good posture, spine in neutral. Take the feet wider than hips and soften the knees, arms relaxed by sides.

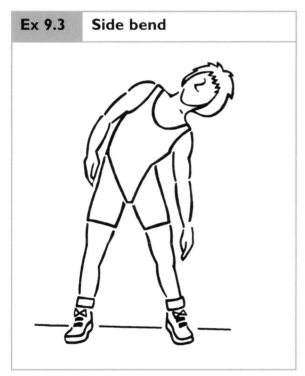

Ex 9.3	Side bend

Action
Keeping the knees soft, draw navel to spine and bend slowly sideways from the waist, reaching down towards the floor. Return to the central position and stand tall. Repeat to alternate sides.

Technique tips
- Bend directly to the side – do not lean forwards or back.
- Keep the weight central throughout – avoid pushing the hips out to the side.
- Bend as far as is comfortable.
- Lift up on the underneath side.
- Lengthen the spine through the centre.
- Keep the movement slow and controlled.

Trunk twist

Purpose: to mobilise the thoracic spine.

Preparation
Stand tall with good posture, spine in neutral. Take the feet wider than hips and soften the knees. Bend the elbows and lift the arms to chest height.

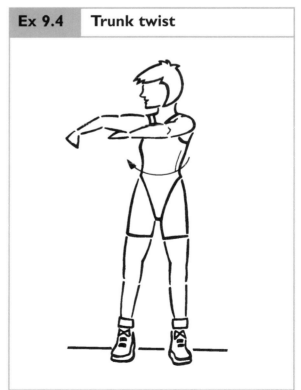

Ex 9.4	Trunk twist

Action
Keeping the knees and hips facing forwards, draw navel to spine, lengthen the torso and slowly turn the upper body around to one side. Return to the central position before repeating to the other side.

Technique tips
- Knees and hips should remain square to the front.
- Keep the shoulder-blades drawn down.
- Pause to check posture between each rotation.
- Lengthen the spine.
- Perform slowly with control.

Caution: Allowing the knees and hips to rotate may be damaging to the knees and lower back.

Hip rotation

Purpose: to loosen and ease tension in the lower back.

Preparation
Stand tall with good posture spine in neutral. Take the feet wider than hips and soften the knees, hands on lower ribcage.

Action
Keeping the knees soft and the spine long, move the hips around in an exaggerated circle to the right. Keep the abdominals lightly held in and avoid arching the back excessively. Perform the desired number of repetitions before changing direction.

Technique tips
- The movement should occur below the hands, avoid moving the upper body.
- Keep the chest lifted and spine long.
- Weight should remain centred between both feet throughout.

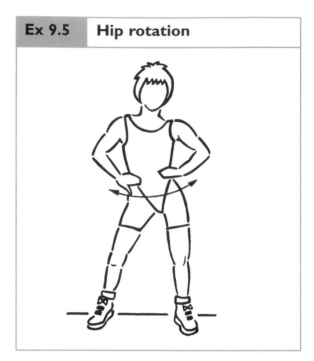

Ex 9.5 | Hip rotation

- Keep the movement controlled and continuous.

Caution: Overemphasising the backward movement may stress the spine.

Heel toe

Purpose: to mobilise the ankles.

Preparation
Stand tall with good posture, neutral spine, hands on hips.

Action
Draw navel to spine as you bend one knee and place the heel of the other foot on the floor in front. Without moving the knee, alternate toe and heel touches to the floor. Perform the desired number of repetitions before repeating on the other side.

Ex 9.6	**Heel toe**

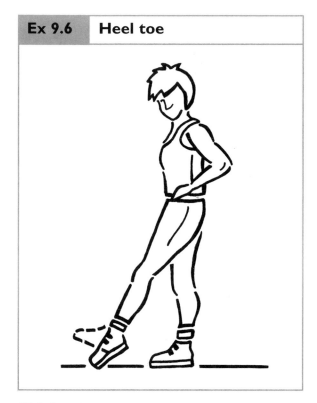

Ex 9.7	**Foot mobility**

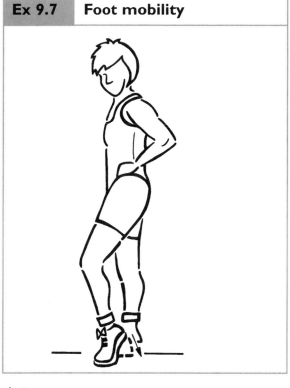

Technique tips
- Ensure the action comes from the ankle and not the knee.
- Pull up out of the supporting hip to avoid pushing out to the side.
- Keep the supporting knee soft and correctly aligned.
- Keep the spine long and the chest open.

Foot mobility

Purpose: to mobilise the ankles and feet and promote the circulation.

Preparation
Stand tall with good posture and feet together, hands on hips. Lift the heel of the right foot off the floor keeping the base of the toe joints pressed down. Keep the hips level and knees soft.

Action
Draw navel to spine as you transfer the weight from right to left foot lifting the arch of the foot as high as possible. Maintain an upright stance throughout. Lift through the supporting hip to avoid rocking and keep the spine long. Continue padding through alternate feet.

Technique tips
- Keep knee aligned over foot.
- Keep equal weight across all toe joints.
- Hinge at the toe joint and emphasise the lift through the arches.
- Avoid rocking the hips from side to side.

Knee bend

Purpose: to mobilise the knees and hips and warm the muscles.

Preparation

Stand tall with good posture, feet wider than hips, comfortably turned out. Place hands on hips.

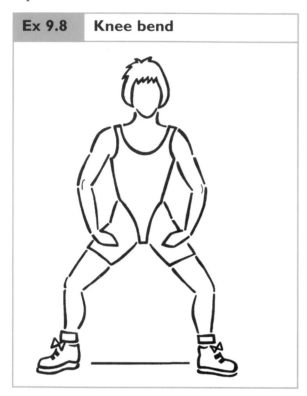

Ex 9.8	Knee bend

Action

Draw navel to spine and bend the knees keeping the heels down and knees aligned with toes. Keep the spine lifted and the head up. Slowly straighten the knees, taking care not to lock them out, maintaining neutral spine. Perform the desired number of repetitions.

Technique tips

- Maintain upright posture and neutral spine throughout.
- Ensure knees move outwards and in line with toes.
- Keep the bend shallow – avoid bending below 90 degrees.

- Focus on drawing the quadriceps up as the knees straighten.

Knee raise

Purpose: to mobilise the hips and knees and warm the muscles.

Preparation

Stand tall with good posture, neutral spine, hands on hips.

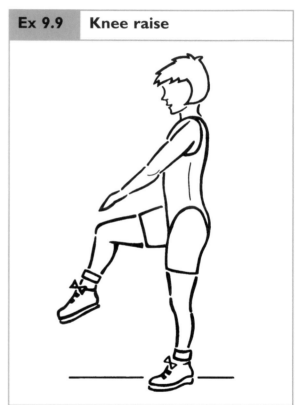

Ex 9.9	Knee raise

Action

Draw navel to spine and lift alternate knees up to a comfortable height in front, keeping the back lifted. Avoid dropping into the supporting hip during the transition. Perform the desired number of repetitions.

Technique tips
- Lift the knee in line with the toes to a comfortable height.
- Replace the foot directly under the hip to prevent the pelvis rocking from side to side.
- Touch the hand to the opposite knee without twisting the torso.
- Keep the chest lifted throughout and avoid dipping towards the knee.
- Maintain navel to spine.

Trunk mobility

Purpose: to open the chest and loosen the upper body.

Preparation
Stand tall with good posture, feet slightly wider than hips and arms relaxed to the sides.

Action
Draw navel to spine, and tilt the pelvis, curling the tailbone under and rounding the upper body forward. Allow the arms to curl forward with the back. Draw navel to spine to lift and lengthen the body back to the upright position, opening the arms out to the side. Perform the desired number of repetitions.

Technique tips
- Relax the head forwards to complete the spinal curl.
- Draw the shoulder-blades down as the spine lengthens.
- Avoid pushing the chest forward on the extension.
- Keep the movement slow and continuous.

Ex 9.10	Trunk mobility

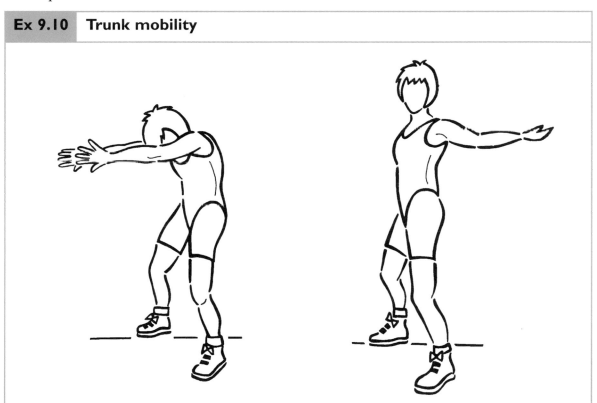

Arm circle

Purpose: to mobilise the shoulder joint.

Preparation
Stand tall with good posture, neutral spine, arms relaxed by sides.

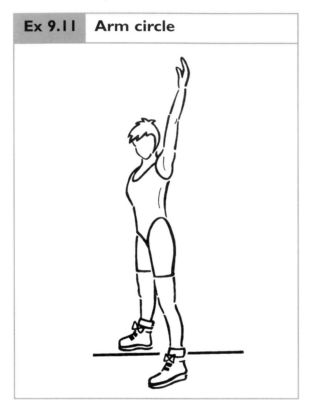

Ex 9.11   Arm circle

Action
Draw navel to spine and take one arm around in a slow circle, keeping the hips and shoulders facing forwards. Make the circle as large as possible. Perform the desired number of repetitions before changing to the other side.

Technique tips
• Keep the arm close to the body throughout.
• Emphasise the full circular movement, paying particular attention to the backward phase.

• Avoid arching the back as the arm moves behind.
• Keep hips and shoulders facing forwards throughout.
• Press the shoulder firmly down on completion of each circle.
• Keep the movement slow and continuous.

Neck mobility

Purpose: to release tension in the neck.

Preparation
Stand tall with good posture in neutral spine. Slide shoulder-blades down and relax arms by sides.

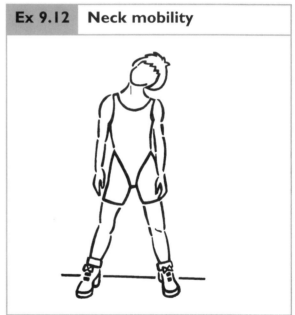

Ex 9.12   Neck mobility

Action
1 Draw navel to spine and, keeping the shoulders relaxed, slowly turn the head to look over the shoulder, pause and return to the centre. Repeat to the other side.
2 Draw navel to spine and tilt the head sidewards, taking ear towards shoulder.

Perform the desired number of repetitions before changing to the other side.

Technique tips
- Keep shoulder-blades sliding down and chest lifted.
- Lengthen through the centre on recovery.
- Perform slowly with control.
- Maintain upright stance.

Standing stretches

Upward reach

Purpose: to stretch the latissimus dorsi muscles and lengthen the spine.

Preparation
Stand tall with good posture, neutral spine, and hands on hips.

Action
Draw navel to spine and reach one arm up, lengthening towards the ceiling. Keep the body weight slightly forwards to avoid arching the back. Pause briefly at the top then lower, keeping the body lifted and tall. Repeat on the other side.

Technique tips
- Draw navel to spine to prevent the back arching.
- Feel a stretch down the side of the body as you reach upwards.
- Keep the shoulders relaxed down.
- Maintain the lengthened spine as you lower the arm.

Calf stretch

Purpose: to stretch gastrocnemius muscle.

Ex 9.13	Upward reach

Ex 9.14	Calf stretch

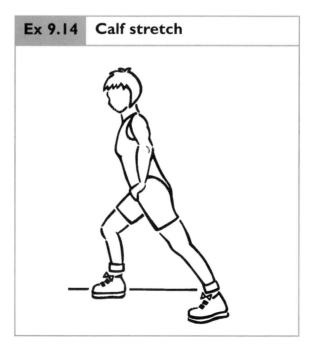

Preparation
Stand tall with good posture, neutral spine, and

hands on hips. Keeping the feet hip-width, take a large step backwards with one foot, keeping both heels down and the feet facing forwards.

Action
Draw navel to spine and bend the front knee, pressing the back heel into the floor with a straight knee. Keep both hips facing forward. Hold for a count of eight and repeat using the other leg.

Technique tips
- Lean slightly forwards with the upper body to maintain a diagonal line from head to heel.
- Keep the chest lifted and open.
- Keep the front knee aligned over ankle.
- Feel the stretch in the bulky part of the calf.
- Move the foot further back for a more intensive stretch.
- Use the wall or a chair for support if required.

Lower calf stretch

Purpose: to stretch the soleus muscle.

Preparation
As for the calf stretch, with feet closer together, weight central.

Action
Draw navel to spine and bend both knees, keeping the back heel on the floor. Move the weight towards the back foot but maintain neutral alignment. Feel a stretch in the lower calf. Hold for a count of eight before repeating on the other leg.

Technique tips
- Keep the shoulders down and the chest open.
- Lift up out of the hips and keep them level.

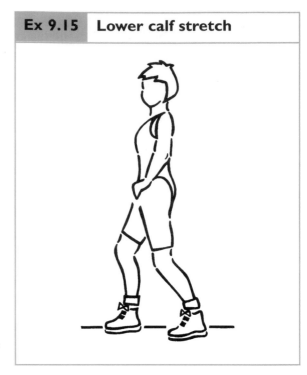

Ex 9.15   Lower calf stretch

- Maintain correct alignment in both knees.
- Adjust the body weight towards the back foot if the stretch is not felt.
- Do not allow the back to arch.
- Use the wall or a chair for support if required.

Quadriceps stretch

Purpose: to stretch the quadriceps muscles.

Preparation
Stand tall with good posture next to a wall or chair, with one hand resting on the support. Bring the outside leg onto the ball of the foot and transfer the weight onto the supporting leg, lifting out of the hip.

Action
Draw navel to spine and bend both knees, lifting the outside knee to take hold of the front

Ex 9.16	Quadriceps stretch

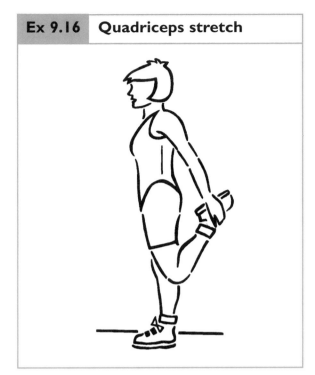

of the foot. Move the knee back until it is under the hip and lift up through the supporting leg keeping the knee soft. Draw the abdominals in again and lengthen the spine. Feel a stretch in the front of the thigh. Hold for a count of eight before repeating on the other leg.

Technique tips
- Maintain neutral spine throughout.
- Hold socks or trousers if it feels uncomfortable to hold the front of the foot.
- Keep the knee pointing downwards and close to the other knee.
- Avoid pulling the foot tightly into the bottom.
- Keep the supporting knee bent.
- If no stretch is experienced move the leg further back and push the hip slightly forward.

Hamstring stretch

Purpose: to stretch the hamstring muscles.

Preparation
Stand tall with good posture, one foot in front of the other. Draw navel to spine and bend both knees, leaning forward and placing both hands in the middle of the back thigh.

Ex 9.17	Hamstring stretch

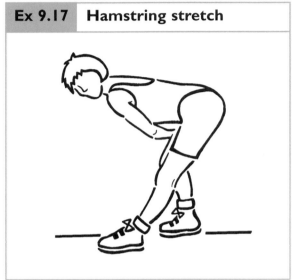

Action
Keeping the abdominals lifted, move the body weight forwards and lift the hips towards the ceiling, slowly straightening the front knee. Feel a stretch in the back of the thigh of the straight leg. Hold for a count of eight before repeating on the other leg.

Technique tips
- Keep supporting knee correctly aligned.
- Avoid sitting back into the stretch – lift the tailbone upwards.
- Maintain abdominal support to prevent the back hyperextending.
- Avoid locking the knee out.
- Keep the spine long and the shoulders down.

Hip flexor stretch

Purpose: to stretch the hip flexor muscles to assist with the maintenance of correct posture.

Preparation

Stand tall with good posture, neutral spine, one hand resting on a support. Keeping the feet hip-width, take a large step backwards with one foot, keeping both feet facing forwards. Lift the back heel off the floor but ensure the weight remains central between both feet.

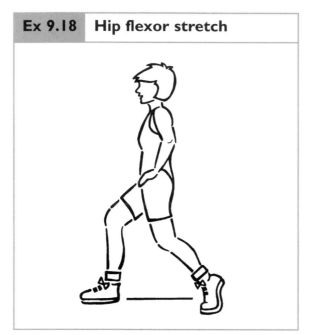

Ex 9.18   Hip flexor stretch

Action

Draw navel to spine to bend the knees and tilt the pelvis to lift the pubic bone upwards. Lengthen the spine and open the chest. Feel a stretch across the front of the hip of the back leg. Hold for a count of eight before repeating on the other leg.

Technique tips
• Keep the knee bend shallow.

• Maintain body weight in the centre of both feet.
• Keep the hips level and facing forward.
• Keep the back lifted but avoid leaning backwards.
• Lengthen through the front of the hip.

Inner thigh stretch

Purpose: to stretch the adductor muscles.

Preparation

Stand tall with good posture, feet as wide as is comfortable and hands on hips. Turn the right foot slightly outwards, keeping the knee aligned, and move the left foot to face straight ahead.

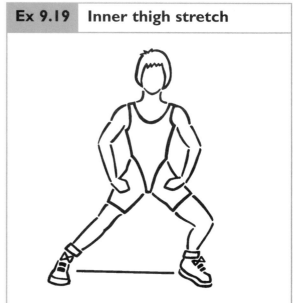

Ex 9.19   Inner thigh stretch

Action

Draw navel to spine and bend the right knee, keeping the left leg straight and both feet flat on the floor. Lengthen the spine and open the chest. Feel a stretch in the inner thigh of the left leg. Hold for a count of eight before repeating on the other side.

Technique tips
- Keep both hips facing forward.
- Take the weight over to the supporting side.
- Keep knee aligned over ankle of bent leg.
- Avoid rolling the ankle or knee of the straight leg.
- If no stretch is felt, draw navel to spine and lift the hips, leaning forward slightly.

Caution: Stop immediately if you experience any discomfort around the pubic bone during this stretch. Try reducing the width of the position, but if it is still uncomfortable omit this stretch from your exercise session.

Chest stretch

Purpose: to stretch the pectoral muscles to assist with correct posture.

Preparation
Stand tall with good posture, hands resting on buttocks, spine in neutral.

Ex 9.20	Chest stretch

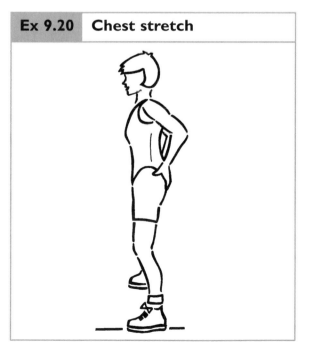

Action
Draw navel to spine and lengthen the elbows away from shoulders, drawing them back as the chest opens. Draw the ribcage down and lengthen the spine. Feel a stretch across the chest and the front of the shoulders. Hold for a count of six – repeat if desired.

Technique tips
- Keep the knees soft.
- Keep the abdominals lightly held to prevent the back arching.
- Draw the ribcage down at the front.
- Lengthen the neck and keep it in line with the spine.

Side stretch

Purpose: to stretch the latissimus dorsi and oblique muscles.

Preparation
Stand tall with good posture, feet slightly wider than hips and hands on hips.

Ex 9.21	Side stretch

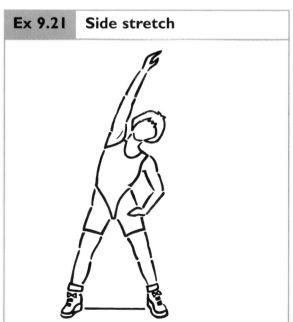

Action

Draw navel to spine and reach the right arm up to the ceiling, lengthening the spine. Continue the lengthening feeling and reach up and over to the left side, sliding the supporting arm down to mid-thigh. Feel a stretch down the right side of body. Hold for a count of six before repeating to the other side.

Technique tips

- Continue the upward reach as the body bends to the side.
- Avoid sinking in the supporting side – keep lengthening away.
- Keep the weight central – avoid pushing the hips out to the side.
- Position the top arm slightly forwards to avoid arching the back.
- Press the shoulders firmly down.
- Keep the abdominals held lightly in to protect the back.

Triceps stretch

Purpose: to lengthen the triceps muscles.

Preparation

Stand tall with good posture.

Action

Draw navel to spine to lift the right arm up to the ceiling, bending the elbow and reaching fingers down between the shoulder-blades. Lift the elbow towards the ceiling with the left hand and ease it gently behind the head. Feel the stretch in the back of the right upper arm. Hold for a count of eight before repeating with the other arm.

Technique tips

- Maintain neutral spine throughout.
- Hinge slightly forward from the hips to prevent the back arching.

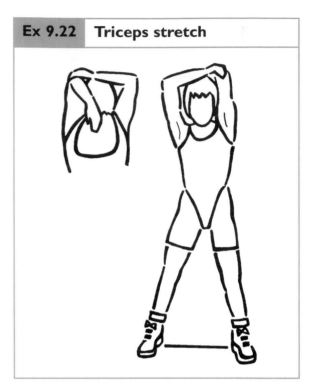

Ex 9.22 | **Triceps stretch**

- Lengthen the elbow away from the shoulder.
- If the back begins to arch, try supporting the stretch from the front rather than overhead.
- Keep the head lifted and in line with the spine.

Standing exercises for muscular strength and endurance

Forward lunge

Purpose: to strengthen the gluteals and quadriceps muscles to assist with bending and lifting.

Preparation

Stand in correct posture, feet hip-width apart and spine in neutral, sideways to a support. Take a large step back with one foot,

Ex 9.23 | Forward lunge

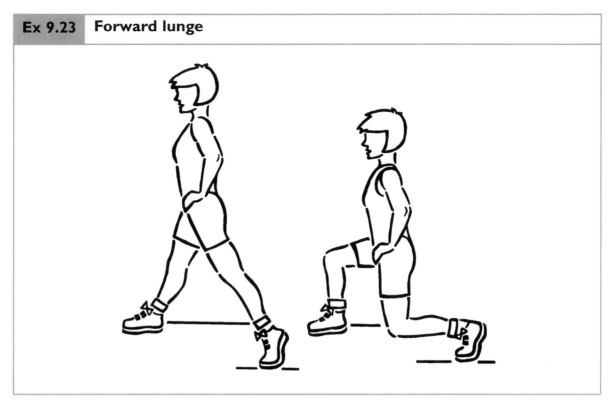

maintaining hip-width and lift the back heel off the floor. Centre the weight between both legs and soften the knees.

Action
Draw navel to spine and bend both knees, lowering the back knee towards the floor. Keep the body weight centred to ensure correct knee/ankle alignment. Return to standing, keeping the spine in neutral and the shoulders down. Perform the desired number of repetitions before changing legs.

Technique tips
• Ensure navel to spine with each repetition.
• Maintain correct postural alignment throughout.
• Keep the front knee aligned over the ankle and back knee under the hip.

• Avoid locking out the knee on return to standing.
• Think of lengthening the spine away from the floor as you bend.
• Perform slowly with control.
• Keep the range of movement small initially and progress to the deeper bend when strength has been gained.

Caution: Stop and check alignment if pain or discomfort is felt in the knees.
  This is an intensive exercise and should commence with low repetitions.

Progression
Once strength has been gained, this exercise can be performed with weights (*see* page 149) or while holding baby!

Calf raise

Purpose: to strengthen the gastrocnemius muscle.

Preparation

Stand facing a wall or chair, in correct posture, feet hip-width apart and spine in neutral. Step back one pace from the wall, resting the hands at shoulder height and looking straight ahead. Centre the weight over the feet and soften the knees.

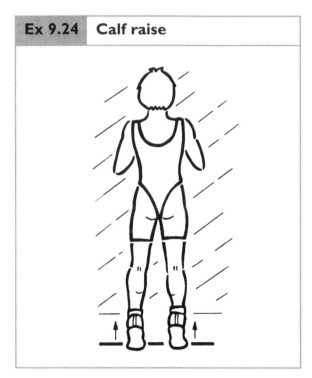

Ex 9.24 Calf raise

Action

Draw navel to spine and rise slowly up onto the toes, keeping feet facing forwards and weight spread evenly between both feet. Lift the arches of the feet and lengthen the spine. Slowly lower the heels to touch lightly on the floor, keeping the weight slightly forwards. Perform the desired number of repetitions.

Technique tips

- Keep the ankles braced to avoid rolling and maintain soft knees.
- Keep the weight spread across the base of all toe joints.
- Lift the arches of the feet as high as possible
- Avoid rolling back on to the heels when lowering.
- Maintain correct spinal alignment throughout.
- Perform slowly and with control.

Progression

Perform this holding baby.

Standing gluteal raise

Purpose: to strengthen the gluteal muscles which aid pelvic stability and assist with bending and lifting.

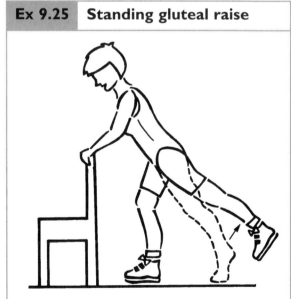

Ex 9.25 Standing gluteal raise

Preparation

Stand two paces back from a wall or chair, facing the support, in correct posture, feet hip-width apart and spine in neutral. Draw navel to spine and lean into the support, hinging at the hips and place hands on the wall at chest height with fingers facing upwards. Straighten one leg out on the floor behind and lengthen it away. Lift through the supporting hip, and soften the knee.

Action
Draw navel to spine and slowly lift the leg up and back, squeezing the buttocks. Keep the upper body forward with both hips square to the wall and supporting knee soft. Lower to the floor keeping the hips level and upper body still. Perform the desired number of repetitions before changing legs.

Technique tips
- The upper body should remain tilted forwards from the hips throughout.
- Keep the hips over the feet.
- Supporting knee soft.
- Shoulder blades sliding down.
- Maintain navel to spine throughout.
- Lift the leg as high as you can without twisting the hips.

Caution: Slow, controlled movements are essential for this exercise to avoid stress to the lower back. Avoid lifting the leg too high as this will cause the back to arch.

Alternative This exercise can also be performed on the floor (*see* page 109).

Standing leg extension

Purpose: to strengthen the quadriceps muscles to aid knee stability.

Preparation
Stand in correct posture, feet hip-width apart and spine in neutral, sideways to a support.

Transfer the weight on to the inside leg and lengthen through the supporting hip. Hold onto the support.

Ex 9.26	**Standing leg extension**

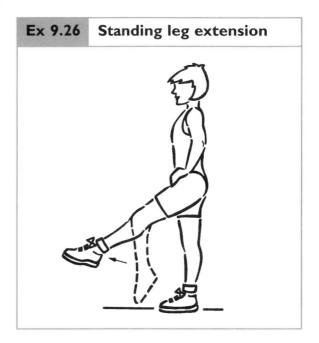

Action
Draw navel to spine and lift the knee of the outside leg. Keeping the thigh lifted, slowly straighten and bend the lower leg, without locking out the knee. Pull up out of the supporting hip to maintain pelvic alignment and keep the spine lengthened. Perform the desired number of repetitions before repeating on the other leg.

Technique tips
- Create a strong, resisted feeling as you straighten the knee.
- Keep the supporting knee soft.
- Maintain good navel to spine contraction and avoid leaning back as the leg straightens.
- Maintain upright posture throughout.
- Perform the exercise slowly and with control.

Wall press-up

Purpose: to strengthen the pectorals and triceps muscles to assist with lifting, carrying and everyday activities.

Preparation
Stand facing a wall or chair, in correct posture, feet hip-width apart and spine in neutral. Step back two paces from the wall and lean into the support, positioning the hands wider than shoulders at the same height, fingers pointing upwards and elbows soft.

Ex 9.27	Wall press-up

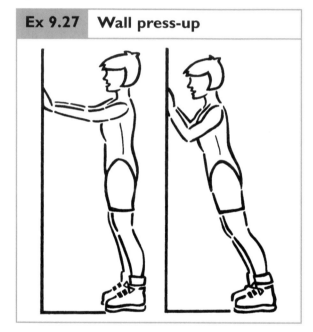

Action
Draw navel to spine, bend the elbows, and lower the upper body towards the wall keeping the spine in neutral. Ensure the bent elbow is in line with the wrist. Slowly straighten the arms and return to the starting position. Perform the desired number of repetitions.

Technique tips
• Maintain correct head alignment.

• Slide shoulder-blades down and lengthen the spine.
• Keep the abdominals lightly held in to maintain spinal alignment.
• Elbows must be directly above wrists – if not, take the hands wider.
• Avoid locking out the elbows on the extension.
• Keep the movement smooth and controlled.

Alternative This exercise can also be performed on the floor (*see* page 108).

Floor exercises for muscular strength and endurance

Bridge with heel raise

Purpose: to strengthen gluteus maximus.

Preparation
Perform the bridge as detailed on page 30.

Action
Hold in the lifted position and transfer the weight onto one side. Draw navel to spine and lift the opposite heel off the floor, keeping the pelvis level. Lower the heel and repeat on the other side. Slowly roll down through the spine to the floor.

Technique tips
• Keep the buttocks lifted but avoid over-squeezing.
• Do not allow the hips to move.
• Draw the ribcage down.
• Keep the spine long.

Progression
Lift the foot just off the floor, keeping the pelvis level and navel to spine.

Alternative
Hold in the lifted bridge position, feet flat and perform scissors or arm circles (*see* pages 19–20). Increasing the length of hold builds up gluteal strength.

Caution Over-squeezing the buttocks and gripping in the hamstrings may induce cramp.

Lying chest press

Purpose: to strengthen the pectoral muscles to help support the breasts and assist with lifting and carrying.

Preparation
Lying supine in neutral alignment with knees bent and feet flat on the floor. Bend the elbows to 90 degrees and lift the arms above the chest with elbows and forearms together, fists lightly clenched.

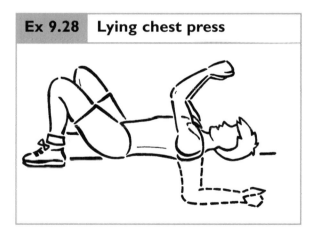

| **Ex 9.28** | **Lying chest press** |

Action
Inhale to prepare and as you exhale draw navel to spine to maintain neutral alignment as the elbows open to the side towards the floor at chest height. Only open the arms as far as neutral can be maintained. Keep the shoulders relaxed and neck long. Inhale, maintaining navel to spine and draw the arms back above

the chest to squeeze the elbows together. Perform the desired number of repetitions.

NB If this arm position pulls the spine out of neutral, keep the elbows just off the floor and draw the ribcage down.

Technique tips
• Keep the elbows at chest height.
• If the breasts feel uncomfortable, keep the elbows slightly apart.
• Press the ribcage into the floor as the arms open.
• Aim to replace the whole arm (forearm and elbow) on the floor each time, maintaining the 90 degree angle.
• Reduce the range if neutral spine is lost.
• Maintain navel to spine, particularly during the opening phase.
• Perform the exercise slowly for maximum effect.
• Breathe throughout.

Press-up

Purpose: to strengthen the pectorals and triceps muscles to assist with lifting, carrying and everyday activities.

Caution: Not to be performed before 6 weeks – see page 21.

Preparation
On hands and knees, in neutral alignment, with knees under hips, hands slightly wider than shoulders and fingers facing forwards. Move the body weight forwards on to your hands, keeping the head correctly aligned.

Action
Draw navel to spine and bend the elbows, slowly lowering the upper body towards the floor. Maintain neutral spine with elbows over

Ex 9.29 Press-up

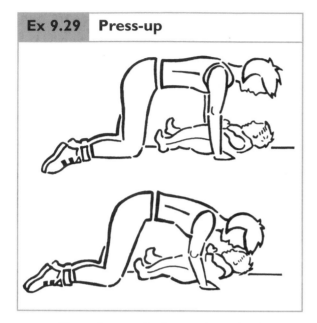

wrists. Keep the weight forwards to slowly push up to the starting position taking care not to lock out the elbows. Perform the desired number of repetitions.

Technique tips
- Keep the head aligned in neutral – do not allow the forehead to drop.
- Aim to touch the nose on the floor between the hands.
- Ensure elbows are over wrists when bending – stop and take the hands wider if necessary.
- Ensure the elbows fully extend but do not lock out.
- Maintain navel to spine and neutral alignment throughout.
- Perform the exercise in a slow, controlled and continuous manner.
- Position baby on the floor in front to encourage the weight forwards.

Progression
- When 20 press-ups can comfortably be performed in this position, move the weight further forwards and repeat with head in front of hands.
- Move the hands and body weight further forwards.

Alternative
If this position is uncomfortable for the knees or tingling/numbness experienced in the fingers, try this exercise standing at the wall (*see* page 106).

Thoracic extension

Purpose: to strengthen lower trapezius and help to improve kyphotic posture.

Preparation
Lie prone (breast comfort permitting) with arms on the floor to the side at shoulder level, elbows bent to 90 degrees and forearms relaxed on the floor. Head relaxed forward on the floor or cushion. Legs together, with toes facing inwards and buttocks relaxed.

Ex 9.30 Thoracic extension

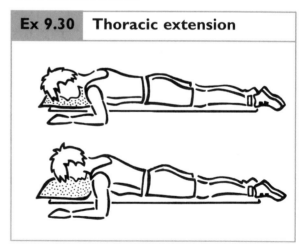

Action
Inhale to prepare, and as you exhale draw navel to spine and press gently down on the forearm lift and lengthen the head and shoulders away from the floor. Inhale to hold,

keeping the abdominals lifted, as you slide the shoulder-blades down. Exhale to lower, lengthening the torso away from the hips. Perform only a small number of repetitions.

Technique tips
- Lift from the lower ribcage.
- Keep the head aligned in neutral – do not drop it back or push the chin forward.
- Extend the spine rather than curling back.
- Keep the abdominals lifted.
- Avoid squeezing the buttocks and pelvic tilting.

Gluteal raise

Purpose: to strengthen the gluteus maximus muscles to aid pelvic stability, postural correction, bending and lifting.

Preparation
On elbows and knees, in neutral alignment, with knees under hips, elbows under shoulders and forearms facing forwards. Draw navel to spine and extend the right leg behind with foot flexed, toes resting on the floor, hips level and facing the floor.

Action
Inhale, and as you exhale draw navel to spine and slowly raise the leg, maintaining neutral alignment and keeping the hips level and square to the floor. Inhale to lower with control, lengthening away from the hip. Perform the desired number of repetitions before repeating on the other leg.

Technique tips
- Ensure navel to spine to maintain correct alignment.
- Lengthen the leg away from the hip, but keep the knee soft.
- Lift through the supporting hip to avoid rolling over on the knee.
- Keep both hip bones facing the floor.
- Lift the leg only as high as good technique permits.
- Perform slowly with control.

Caution: Slow, controlled movements are essential for this exercise to avoid stress to the lower back. Avoid lifting the leg too high as this will cause the back to arch.

Alternative If this position is uncomfortable for

| **Ex 9.31** | **Gluteal raise** |

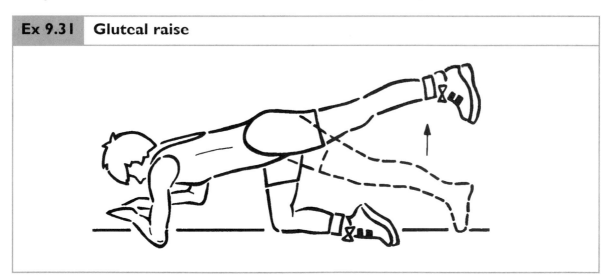

Ex 9.32   Outer thigh raise

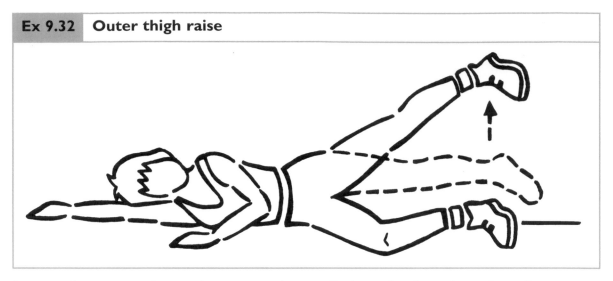

knees or breasts, try the standing version (*see* page 104).

Outer thigh raise

Purpose: to strengthen the gluteus medius and minimus muscles to aid pelvic stability.

Preparation
Side lying with underneath leg bent, knee slightly forward and top leg straight. Rest head on the underneath arm and try to lift the waistband away from the floor. Flex the top foot and rotate the leg forwards so the side of the thigh faces the ceiling and the toes are angled downwards. Lean slightly forwards on to the top arm which is resting on the floor, spine in neutral.

Action
Inhale to prepare and as you exhale, draw navel to spine and slowly lift the top leg, keeping the hip rotated forwards and the knee soft. Lift as high as the joint permits. Inhale to lower slowly with control, keeping the waistband lifted away from the floor.

Perform the desired number of repetitions before repeating on the other leg.

Technique tips
- Lengthen the leg away from the hip.
- Lift the waistband away from the floor.
- Maintain neutral alignment.
- Perform slowly and carefully – don't be tempted to throw the leg up.
- Bend the top knee if it feels uncomfortable.
- Create a feeling of resistance in the muscle as the leg lowers.
- Avoid overflexing the foot and creating tension in the lower leg.
- Keep the hip rotated forward – allowing it to drop back will involve the quadriceps and hip flexors rather than the intended muscles.
- Keep the top shoulder drawn down.

Progression
Keep the toes just off the floor on lowering.

Caution: Stop immediately if pain is experienced in the front or back of the pelvis. If it simply feels uncomfortable in these areas, check your technique and try again. Stop if discomfort persists.

Ex 9.33	Side lying knee raise

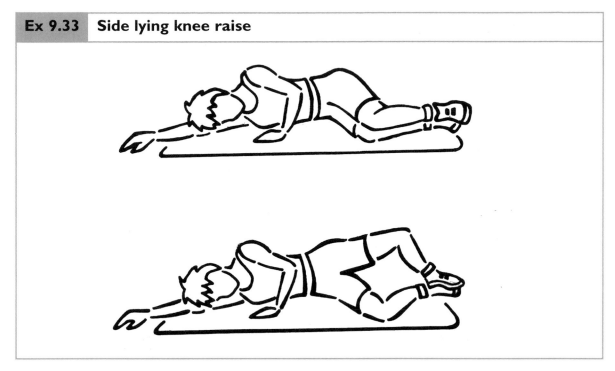

Side lying knee raise

Purpose: to strengthen gluteus medius to assist with pelvic stability.

Preparation
Side lying with legs together and knees bent to 45 degrees with heels together. Underneath arm extended beneath head, top arm relaxed on the floor in front, with shoulder drawn down. Spine in neutral.

Action
Inhale to prepare, and as you exhale draw navel to spine and lift the top knee, keeping feet together and rotating at the hip. Do not allow the pelvis to rock backwards. Inhale to lower with control.

Technique tips
- Maintain neutral spine.
- Keep the hips vertically stacked throughout.
- Lift only as far as you can maintain pelvic alignment.
- Feel the buttock muscles drawing the leg around.
- Keep the top shoulder drawn down.

Inner thigh raise

Purpose: to strengthen the adductor muscles to aid pelvic stability.

Caution: This exercise should not be attempted if you are experiencing pain or discomfort around the pubic bone.

Preparation
Side lying in neutral alignment with head resting on the underneath arm. Bend the top leg and place the knee on a couple of cushions on the floor to maintain knee/hip alignment. Straighten the underneath leg and ensure the

Ex 9.34 | Inner thigh raise

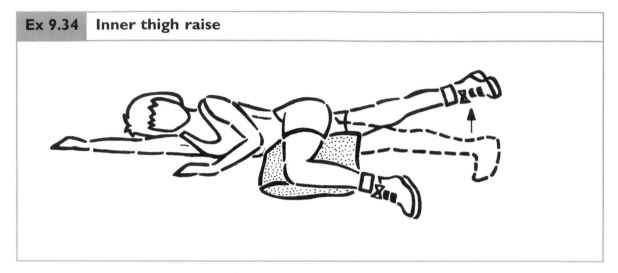

inner thigh faces upwards. Rest the top hand on the floor in front for support with shoulder relaxed down. Lengthen the spine and try to lift the waistband away from the floor.

Action
Inhale to prepare, and as you exhale draw navel to spine and lift the underneath leg towards the ceiling, keeping the inner thigh uppermost and the knee soft. Inhale to lower with control, keeping the upper body relaxed down. Perform the desired number of repetitions before repeating on the other leg.

Technique tips
- Maintain neutral alignment throughout.
- Feel the waistband lifting away from the floor as navel draws into spine.
- Lengthen the leg away from the hip.
- Soften the underneath knee more if discomfort is felt in the knee joint.
- Avoid overflexing the foot and creating tension in the lower leg.
- Perform the exercise slowly and with control.
- Lower the top knee if discomfort is felt in the sacroiliac joint.

Progression
To make the exercise harder, do not let the foot touch the floor on lowering.

Cool-down stretches

Lying body reach
Purpose: to lengthen the body.

Preparation
Lying supine, straighten the legs out along the floor one at a time, and relax the arms on the floor above the head. If this causes the back to arch, bend the knees a little.

Action
Inhale and extend the arms and legs as far away from the centre as is comfortable, reaching from fingers to toes. Exhale to hold the new position, drawing navel to spine and pressing the ribcage into the floor. Perform a limited number of repetitions.

Technique tips
- Pointing the toes may induce cramp – perform with flexed feet if susceptible.

Ex 9.35 Lying body reach

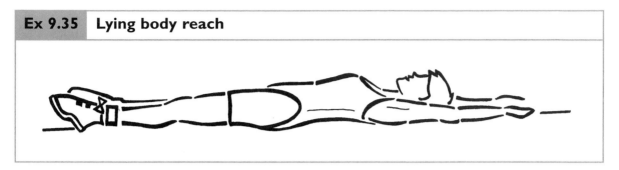

- Keep the extended feeling on release.
- Avoid hyperextending the spine.

Caution: Caesarean deliveries may be very hesitant with this stretch but should be reassured and encouraged to perform slowly. It is particularly valuable as it helps to lengthen the scar tissue.

Lying hamstring stretch

Purpose: to lengthen the hamstring muscles.

Preparation
Lying supine in neutral alignment, with knees bent and feet flat on the floor.

Ex 9.36 Lying hamstring stretch

Action
Lift one knee up and hold the back of the thigh with both hands. Draw navel to spine and begin to straighten the knee until a stretch is felt in the back of the thigh. Support both the upper and lower leg if desired. Relax and hold the stretch for a count of 10. Lower the leg to the floor and repeat on the other side.

Technique tips
- Keep the buttocks on the floor throughout.
- Keep the knee aligned with the hip.
- Keep the leg aligned with the same shoulder.
- Aim to straighten the knee rather than drawing in closer with a bent knee.
- Ease slowly into the stretch and do not bounce.
- Relax the upper body.
- Do not attempt to stretch beyond the normal range.
- If the leg begins to tremble, lower the leg and begin the stretch again – slowly.

Alternatives
- Hold a band around the sole of the foot and use it to draw the leg in.
- Perform in a seated position (*see* page 116).

Progression
Straighten the underneath leg to increase the intensity – approach cautiously as this may pull the lower back.

Lying gluteal stretch

Purpose: to lengthen the gluteus medius and minimus muscles.

Preparation
Lying supine in neutral alignment, with knees bent and feet flat on the floor. Bend the right knee and cross the ankle over the left thigh, just above the knee.

Ex 9.37	Lying gluteal stretch

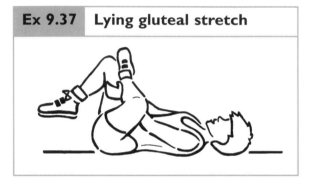

Action
Take hold of the left thigh with one hand either side, draw navel to spine and lift the leg off the floor bringing the knee in towards the chest. Keep the right leg in position with the knee out to the side and ensure the ankle is well supported on the thigh. Feel a stretch in the outer thigh of the right leg. Hold for a count of 10, breathing throughout. Repeat on the other leg.

Technique tips
- Do not allow the ankle of the crossed leg to roll outwards – take the foot further across the thigh.
- Keep the knee out to the side.
- Lengthen the neck and keep the shoulders down.
- Keep elbows soft.
- Maintain navel to spine.
- Breathe throughout.

Caution: Caesarean deliveries may find this stretch pulls on the scar.

Alternative
Perform in a seated position (*see* page 116).

Piriformis stretch

Purpose: to stretch the deep buttock muscles. This may be helpful for women suffering from sciatica.

Ex 9.38	Piriformis stretch

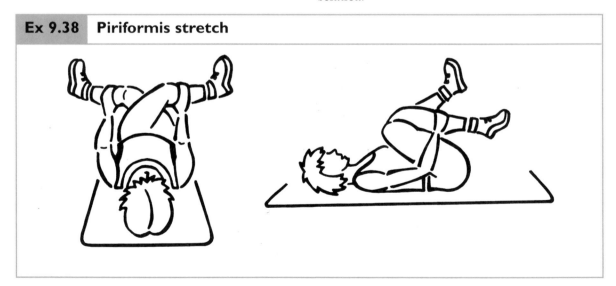

Preparation
Lying supine with knees lifted into chest. Draw navel to spine and cross right knee over left.

Action
Use both arms to draw the back knee towards the chest. Feel a deep stretch radiating across the right buttock. Hold for a count of eight. Repeat slowly on the other side.

Technique tips
- Pull firmly with the arms to draw both knees towards the chest to secure the stretch.
- If no stretch is felt: hold the right calf with the left hand and the left calf with the right hand, and, keeping knees into chest, draw both lower legs out to the side.
- Keep the head relaxed down.
- Keep the hips square – avoid rolling to one side.

Side circle

Purpose: to release the upper body and stretch the pectorals.

Preparation
Side lying with knees bent up together to 45 degrees. Both arms extended in front at chest height, with palms together, head relaxed on the floor. Spine in neutral and shoulders relaxed.

Action
Inhale and circle the top arm around above the head, as close to the floor as possible. Follow the hand with the head. As you exhale, draw navel to spine and continue the circle around to the other side, turning the head to look behind. Pause with both arms open to the side just below shoulder height and hips stacked, continuing to breathe. To return: inhale to prepare, and as you exhale draw navel to spine

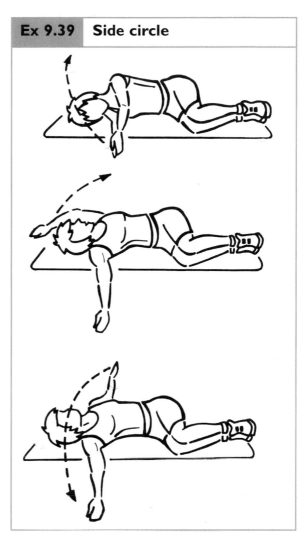

Ex 9.39   Side circle

and reach the arm up and over the chest in a straight line to return to start position.

Technique tips
- Keep fingers in contact with the floor for as long as possible.
- Reach the fingers away from the shoulder.
- Release the neck as it turns.
- Pause and release in an open chest stretch.
- Initiate the return with the abdominals by drawing ribs across to opposite hips.

- Keep the hips stacked – avoid rolling the pelvis backwards.

Caution: Rotation in the pelvis may stress the sacroiliac joints. This exercise should be avoided if sacroiliac problems exist.

Seated hamstring stretch

Purpose: to lengthen the hamstring muscles.

Preparation
Seated on the floor with one leg straight out in front, knee soft, and the other leg bent to the side in a comfortable position. Lift up onto sit bones and use the arms on the floor behind to support the back in neutral alignment.

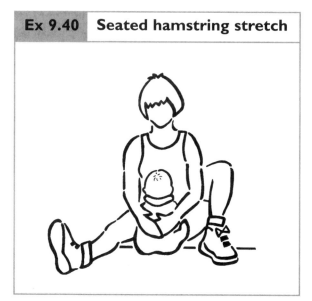

Ex 9.40 **Seated hamstring stretch**

Action
Draw navel to spine and press down onto the hands to lengthen the spine. Slowly incline the body forwards until you feel a stretch in the back of the straight leg. Keep the knees and toes of the straight leg facing up. Hold for a count of 10 before repeating on the other leg.

Technique tips
- Maintain neutral alignment – avoid rolling back off the sit bones.
- Keep the spine long and chest lifted.
- Keep the knee soft on the stretching leg.
- If neutral alignment can be maintained, place the hands on the floor in front.
- This stretch can be performed supporting baby in front.
- If no stretch is experienced, push down on the hands and lift the buttocks slightly back, keeping the heel in place.

Seated gluteal stretch

Purpose: to lengthen the gluteus medius and minimus muscles.

Preparation
Seated on the floor with one leg straight out in front, knee soft, the other bent over the straight leg with foot flat on the floor, close to the other leg. Lift up onto sit bones and use the arms on the floor behind to support the back in neutral alignment.

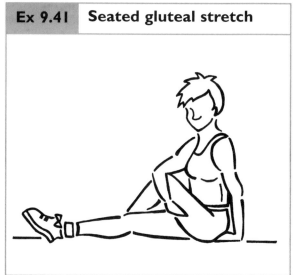

Ex 9.41 **Seated gluteal stretch**

Action

Draw navel to spine and wrap the opposite arm around the bent knee, gently hugging the knee towards the chest. Keeping the spine lengthened and both buttocks firmly on the floor, gently rotate the upper body away from the lifted knee. Feel a stretch in the side of the crossed leg. Hold for a count of eight before repeating on the other leg.

Technique tips
- Cradle the knee into chest with the elbow and forearm.
- Lengthen the spine away from sit bones.
- Maintain neutral alignment.
- Abdominals must be drawn in prior to rotating.
- Move the foot closer to hip if the stretch is not felt.
- Keep both buttocks firmly on the floor.
- Avoid the rotation if breasts are uncomfortable or perform lying supine (*see* page 114).
- Breathe throughout.

Seated adductor stretch

Purpose: to lengthen the adductor muscles.

Preparation

Seated on the floor with soles of the feet together and knees open to the side. Lift up onto sit bones and use the arms on the floor behind to support the back in neutral alignment.

Action

Using the arms behind for support, draw navel to spine and slide the buttocks in towards the heels until a stretch is felt in the inner thighs. Relax the knees, and hold for a count of 10, continuing to breathe.

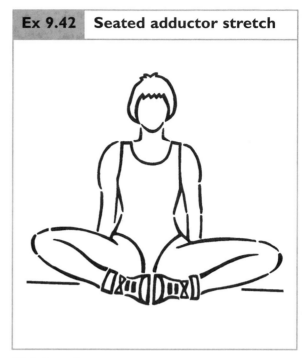

Ex 9.42 **Seated adductor stretch**

Technique tips
- Push the body weight slightly forwards with the hands.
- Avoid locking out the elbows.
- Lengthen the spine away from sit bones.
- Maintain neutral alignment with navel to spine.
- Keep both buttocks firmly in the floor.
- Place your hands on the floor in front if this is more comfortable.
- Do not attempt to push too far with this stretch.

Caution: Stop immediately if pain is experienced on the pubic bone.

Seated chest stretch

Purpose: to lengthen the pectorals and improve posture.

Ex 9.43	Seated chest stretch

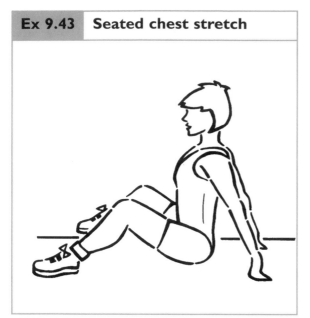

Seated triceps stretch

Purpose: to lengthen the triceps muscles.

Preparation
Seated on the floor with legs in a comfortable position, spine in neutral and lengthened away from floor.

Ex 9.44	Seated triceps stretch

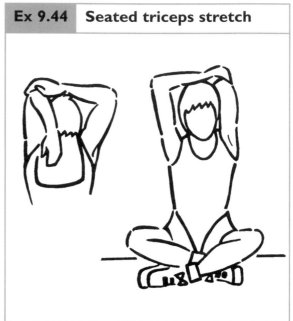

Preparation
Seated on the floor with legs in a comfortable position, spine in neutral and lengthened away from floor. Without taking the weight backwards, rest the fingertips on the floor behind the buttocks.

Action
Draw navel to spine and open the elbows back as shoulder blades squeeze together. Draw the ribcage down to prevent the chest lifting and maintain neutral spine. Feel a stretch across the chest and the front of the shoulders. Hold for a count of six, breathing throughout.

Technique tips
- Keep the weight on the buttocks, avoid leaning back onto the arms.
- Lengthen the spine away from sit bones.
- Open the chest but do not lift it.
- Draw the ribcage and shoulder-blades down.
- Maintain neutral alignment and navel to spine.
- Avoid locking out the elbows.

Action
Draw navel to spine to lift the right arm up to the ceiling, bending the elbow and reaching fingers down between the shoulder blades. Lift the elbow towards the ceiling with the left hand and ease it gently behind the head. Feel the stretch in the back of the right upper arm. Hold for a count of eight before repeating with the other arm.

Technique tips
- Maintain neutral spine throughout.
- Hinge slightly forward from the hips to prevent the back arching.

- Lengthen the elbow away from the shoulder.
- If the back begins to arch, try supporting the stretch from the front rather than overhead.
- Keep the head lifted and in line with the spine.

Alternative

This stretch may be more comfortable performed in a standing position.

Seated upper back stretch

Purpose: to lengthen the trapezius muscles.

NB Postural changes may result in these muscles lengthening and tightening. Trapezius stretching is still very relevant, although great emphasis is not placed on it.

Preparation

Seated on the floor with legs in a comfortable position, spine in neutral and lengthened away from floor. Lift the elbows out to the side and

bring the arms around in front, each hand taking hold of the opposite arm just below the elbow.

Action

Keeping the arms bent, draw navel to spine, perform a pelvic tilt and curve the back, pressing the shoulders forwards and curling the head. Feel a stretch across the top of the back. Hold for a count of six, breathing throughout.

Technique tips

- Lift the elbows to the side first when moving into position; this opens up the back and makes the stretch more effective.
- Draw the shoulder blades down.
- Ensure navel to spine occurs before rolling off sit bones.
- Avoid sinking on the pelvic tilt, lengthen the tail bone under.
- Keep the elbows bent.
- Keep shoulders over hips – avoid leaning forwards from the hips.
- Allow the head to complete the spine curl.

Seated side stretch

Purpose: to lengthen latissimus dorsi and oblique muscles.

Preparation

Seated on the floor with legs in a comfortable position, spine in neutral and lengthened away from floor. Hands resting to the side on the floor.

Action

Draw navel to spine and reach the right arm up to the ceiling, lengthening the spine. Continue the lengthening feeling and reach up and over to the left side, sliding the supporting hand further away from the body. Feel a stretch down the right side of body. Hold for a count of six before repeating to the other side.

Ex 9.45	Seated upper back stretch

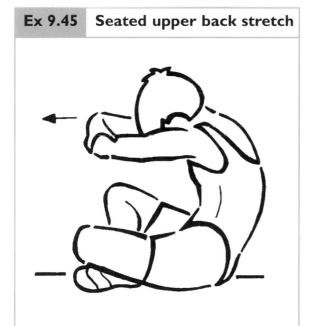

Ex 9.46	Seated side stretch

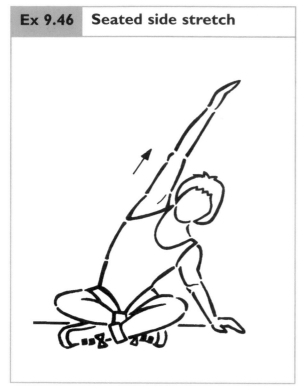

Technique tips

- Continue the upward reach as the body bends to the side.
- Avoid sinking in the supporting side – keep lengthening away.
- Keep both buttocks firmly on the floor.
- Position the top arm slightly forwards to avoid arching the back.
- Press the shoulders firmly down.
- Keep the abdominals held lightly in to protect the back.

Seated neck stretch

Purpose: to lengthen the muscles in the neck and release tension.

Preparation

Seated on the floor with legs in a comfortable position, spine in neutral and lengthened away

Ex 9.47	Seated neck stretch

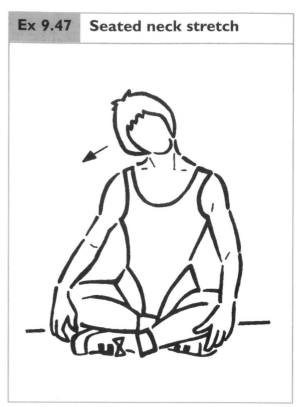

from floor. Hands resting to the side on the floor.

Action

Keeping the spine long, draw navel to spine and tilt the head to the right side, taking the ear towards your shoulder. Press the shoulders down and feel a stretch down the left side of your neck. Pause and return to the centre. Repeat on the other side, breathing throughout.

Technique tips

- Lengthen the spine away from sit bones.
- Draw the ribcage and shoulder-blades down.
- Maintain neutral alignment and navel to spine.
- Ensure the movement comes only from the neck.

Ex 9.48	**Relaxation**

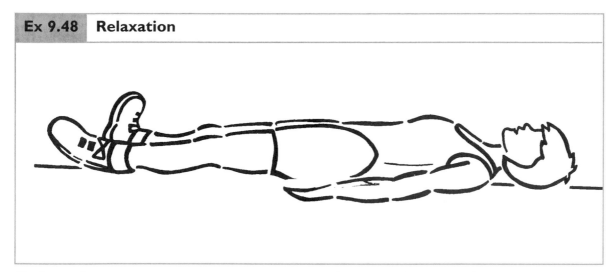

Relaxation

Purpose: to release tension and rest the body.

Preparation
Lying supine with cushions under the head and thighs, if desired. Choose a comfortable position for the head and close your eyes. Feel the body well supported by the floor and the cushions.

Action
Roll the legs and feet outwards from the hips and let go. Roll the arms out from the shoulders so the palms face the ceiling. Breathe gently in and out in your own time and try to relax a little more with each breath out. Feel yourself sinking into the support. Focus your thoughts on something that makes you feel calm and relaxed. Remain in this position for as long as you can.

Recovery
Give yourself adequate time to recover when the relaxation is over. Open your eyes and slowly readjust to your environment. Draw navel to spine, bend your knees one at a time and put feet flat on the floor. With knees and feet together, roll carefully over onto one side and rest in this position for a short while. When you feel ready to get up, slowly push yourself up with your hands and move into a sitting position. If possible, rest in this position and perform some of the mobility moves from the beginning of this chapter (e.g. shoulder rolls, neck mobility, side bends), before moving to standing. For a more detailed relaxation session, see Chapter 13.

Upward reach

Purpose: to stretch and refresh.

Preparation
Stand tall with good posture, neutral spine, hands relaxed by sides with palms up.

Action
Inhale and lengthen the arms away from the shoulder as they circle up to the ceiling, drawing navel to spine. Maintain neutral alignment as the arms lift. Exhale to rotate the shoulder and lower the arms, pressing palms to the floor. Perform several times.

Ex 9.48	Upward reach

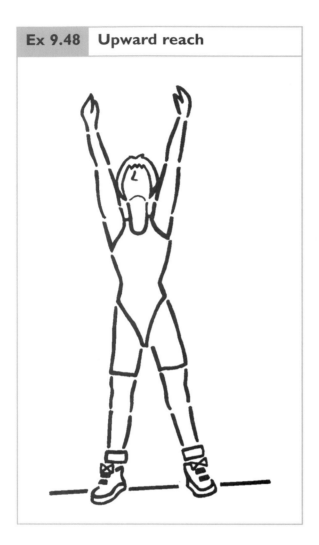

Technique tips

- Slide the shoulder-blades down as the arms lift.
- Keep the arms slightly forward to maintain neutral.
- Draw down in the ribcage to avoid the chest lifting.
- Extend the arms away from the shoulders throughout.
- Maintain the length in the spine as the arms lower.

CARDIOVASCULAR TRAINING

10

Benefits of cardiovascular training

Regular cardiovascular exercise of the appropriate intensity, duration and type is extremely beneficial in assisting postnatal recovery. Increased circulation promotes blood flow through varicose veins and aids resorption of excess fluid retained as a result of pregnancy. The improved efficiency of the heart and lungs to transport and utilise oxygen and the increased endurance of the leg muscles will help to make everyday tasks much easier to perform. Cardiovascular exercise is helpful for reducing weight gained during pregnancy and can also be therapeutic for reducing stress and anxiety by assisting with the dispersal of adrenalin (*see* page 162).

Implications

Joints and relaxin

The continuing effects of relaxin on joint stability following the birth have implications for the type of exercise selected. These effects may be prolonged if breastfeeding continues. Low-impact activities are recommended and correct joint alignment essential. Excessive movement of the pelvis, particularly during weight-bearing activities, may stress the symphysis pubis and sacroiliac joints which may aggravate a previous condition or develop a new problem. Increased Q angle of the femur, occurring during pregnancy as a result of pelvic widening, may continue and result in inverted knee alignment, which will stress the patella. Knees are particularly vulnerable during stepping or cycling with the repeated flexion and extension, and the length of time spent on these activities should be considered in proportion to the amount of bending required for everyday babycare. Ankles are also vulnerable to the repetitive stress of jogging or walking and there is an increased risk of ankle misalignment or twisting, particularly on uneven surfaces. Correct posture and exercise technique must be maintained at all times and the duration of the session carefully considered in relation to this.

Pelvic floor

High-impact activities are extremely stressful to the pelvic floor and contra-indicated with the presence of stress incontinence. These muscles are already weak following delivery, and impact may weaken them further and predispose them to this unpleasant condition. Furthermore, decreased ligament support for the pelvic organs may increase the risk of prolapse, a more serious condition which could require surgical repair. Comfort for the perineum should be considered when selecting seated cardiovascular equipment as this may restrict the choice and limit participation, i.e. the saddle of an upright bike is more likely to cause discomfort than the seat of a recumbent bike. Pelvic floor contractions should be encouraged during every activity. Navel to spine will also incur some pelvic floor response (*see* Chapter 3).

Abdominals

The weak, stretched abdominal musculature will have reduced stabilising effects on the spine during whole body movements. TrA must engage to stabilise the spine and this workload increases with co-ordinated arm and leg actions which require internal and external obliques to co-contract to prevent pelvic rotation. Such demands are further increased with speed. It is essential that some degree of abdominal core training has been undertaken prior to commencement of the more demanding cardiovascular work.

Breasts

High-impact activities are unsuitable for breastfeeding as the breasts will feel very heavy and uncomfortable and may leak with excessive movement. They should always be well supported during exercise. Low-impact cardiovascular exercise is recommended but should not involve a large amount of arm work. Movements that bump or squeeze the breasts will be uncomfortable and need adaptation – even when walking, the relaxed arm swinging action may rub against the breasts. Activities such as the rower and cross-trainer that involve a lot of upper body work, may also encourage milk flow. Intensity is particularly relevant to breastfeeding as exercising too vigorously may cause dehydration and fatigue and reduce the amount of milk available for the next feed. Also, the increased production of lactic acid during very intense training may give post-exercise breast milk a sour taste. Increased levels of lactic acid in the milk may remain for at least 90 minutes. Exercising at a gentle to moderate intensity and taking regular sips of water during the workout is strongly recommended.

Weight loss

Weight loss is a priority for most postnatal women and is often the principal reason for undertaking cardiovascular exercise. Losing weight is simply a matter of burning more calories than are consumed each day, therefore exercise of any intensity will help. However, activities undertaken at a comfortably challenging level will not only be safer but can be continued for a longer duration and therefore utilise additional calories. Low to moderate intensity (50–70% MHR) for 20–30 minutes is recommended. Breastfeeding does, however, require additional calories to ensure an adequate supply of milk so if excessive training is undertaken, and calories burned continually exceeds calories consumed, there is a strong possibility that the resulting weight loss will significantly reduce or even halt milk production.

Considerations

How often should cardiovascular exercise be undertaken?

In the early weeks following the birth it may be difficult to find time for specific exercise so it is important to have parts of the day that are more active than others. Daily walks with the baby are an ideal introduction to regular gentle exercise and can quite easily be integrated into the routine of an organised new mum. If undertaken on a regular basis the duration need only be 10 minutes. Less frequent sessions would require a longer duration in order to gain similar benefits. A previously fit woman, on the other hand, may attempt to return immediately to her pre-pregnancy training regime in a desperate attempt to regain her previous shape. This should be discouraged as the effects of pregnancy and delivery will have taken a greater toll on her body than may be realised, and there is a strong possibility that overexertion in the early weeks will impede recovery. Cardiovascular training should build up to the optimum three sessions per week but should not exceed five. The risks involved with more frequent exercise may outweigh the potential benefits. Rest is essential for a new mum and a period of relaxation should be structured into the day in exactly the same way that exercise is.

What intensity is recommended?

Similar aerobic benefits can be achieved by performing high-intensity/short-duration exercise as can be achieved by low-intensity/long-duration exercise but the latter is a much more suitable option. Gentle to moderate intensity is recommended in the early weeks, progressing to a moderate level as energy increases. Heart rate should be maintained at 50–70% MHR for the duration of the activity. If equipment is used, exercise intensity may be monitored automatically by the machine, which provides detailed information of exercising heart rate, calories burned, etc. If heart rate monitoring is not used, the 'talk test' provides a realistic guide to exercising within the comfort zone and breathing should be comfortable and rhythmical throughout. If using RPE the score should be between 'light' and 'somewhat hard' and one should feel warm and slightly breathless. (*See* Appendix for more details.)

How long should the session last?

Commencing with 10 minutes of cardiovascular work (not including warm-up and cool-down) should be sufficient to gain small benefits if performed a few times a week. Less frequent sessions would require a longer duration. This could gradually increase to 20 and up to 30 minutes providing the intensity remains gentle to moderate. Varying the intensity between these two levels and incorporating periods of rest into the workout will prevent it becoming too demanding. A further factor for consideration is local muscular endurance, which will shorten the duration if fatigue sets in. Continuing over an extended period of time also increases the risk of injury to the joints and pelvic floor.

Types of cardiovascular training

A variety of cardiovascular activities is available, some more suitable than others for postnatal women. The optimum three sessions a week should ideally comprise different activities, i.e. a brisk walk with the baby, a swim and a session on the bike. Activities should be introduced individually on separate occasions so that, should problems develop, the cause can be more easily identified. Studio-based cardiovascular activities are discussed in Chapter 12.

Walking

This is an excellent activity as it can easily be incorporated into a new lifestyle with baby. A brisk walk around the park needs no special equipment apart from a suitable sturdy pushchair, and can be undertaken at any convenient time. The main consideration is the height of the pushchair handle in relation to spinal alignment; a stooped position may be adopted if the handle is too low, particularly when speed increases or when terrain varies. Walking without baby offers a potentially better workout as the upper body can be employed in the activity and correct postural alignment maintained. Spinal alignment should be corrected if heavy breasts pull the upper back forwards, although an over-compensated, leaning back position will increase stress on the lumbar spine. Excessive pelvic movement may occur when the pace increases as the body weight rocks from side to side; this should be avoided to prevent sacroiliac and symphysis pubis misalignment. Outdoor walking offers the benefits of sunlight; which provides vitamin D, essential for the absorption of calcium (*see* page 46), fresh air and adequate cooling for the body. Variable terrain walking provides intensity changes, but may increase the risk of incorrect joint alignment. Adherence to correct technique is vital, particularly when speed increases and pelvic movement becomes more accentuated. The following key points apply to treadmill or outdoor walking:

- Maintain correct postural alignment and walk tall.
- Draw navel to spine frequently.
- Take long, comfortable strides.
- Use a heel-toe action to roll through the foot.
- Push off from the big toe and lift the arch of the foot.
- Keep knees aligned – avoid rolling in.
- Keep the hips level and avoid dipping from side to side.
- Relax the shoulders and open the chest.
- Allow the arms to swing naturally by the sides.

Caution: If pain is experienced on the pubic bone or in the groin this activity should be stopped and an alternative method of training adopted.

Jogging

Jogging raises more concerns than walking as stress to the joints is increased twofold. High-impact incline training further increases joint stress, threefold uphill and fourfold downhill. This is compounded by reduced joint stability, which may continue for many weeks after delivery. Key areas of concern are:

- Dropped metatarsal arches, as a result of relaxin, may cause a flat-footed strike which will not absorb impact in the correct way.
- Relaxin effects may reduce stability of the ankle joint and increase vulnerability to sprains.
- Increased Q angle of the femur may prevent adoption of correct knee alignment.
- Reduced pelvic stability may allow an excessive rolling hip action.

The pelvic floor is subjected to a high degree of stress during high-impact activities which may further weaken the area and increase the risk of a prolapse. Large breasts will feel extremely uncomfortable while jogging and may leak with the excessive movement.

Outdoor running requires a greater stabilising role from TrA; variable terrain is more likely to throw the body off balance and the abdominal musculature needs to respond quickly to prevent injury. Correct jogging action plays a vital role in reducing these risk factors by keeping the stride low to the ground and ensuring a heel-toe action for maximal shock absorption.

Key points:
- Wear a bra that provides sufficient support for the breasts and reduces the bounce.
- Select appropriate footwear, preferably a running shoe, that is designed to absorb the shock through the heel and support the ankle joint.
- Maintain correct neutral alignment and run tall.
- Draw navel to spine frequently.
- Take easy, comfortable strides.

- Aim for a heel strike directly under the knee.
- Use a heel-toe action to roll through the foot.
- Push off from the big toe and lift the arch of the foot.
- Keep knees aligned – avoid rolling in.
- Relax the shoulders and open the chest.
- Bend the elbows and keep them close to the body.
- Allow a gentle forwards and backwards arm motion.

Caution: Avoid excessive pelvic movement; avoid leaning back; support the breasts adequately.

Recumbent bike

Cycling is particularly suitable for postnatal women as the bodyweight is supported, reducing stress on the bones and joints. The recumbent bike, as opposed to the upright bike, is more appropriate as the seated position provides support for the spine whereas the forward leaning position of an upright bike will increase the thoracic curve already present from breast growth. Additionally, the seat is much more comfortable than the saddle of an upright bike, which may be quite painful for a sore perineum. The raised leg position of the recumbent bike is particularly beneficial as it aids circulation and venous return. The recumbent position, however, relies very heavily on the quadriceps and hamstrings and local muscle fatigue may limit duration. Seat positioning is crucial to avoid stress to the pelvis and knees; one that is too far forward may place excessive strain on the knees and one that is too far back requires the pelvis to shift from side to side in order to extend the knee effectively. A comfortable seated position should allow the knees to be extended but not locked out and the pelvis should remain still. Studio cycling is discussed in Chapter 12.

Key points:
- Maintain correct neutral alignment and sit tall.
- Draw navel to spine throughout.
- Keep knees aligned – avoid rolling in.
- Keep pelvis still throughout.
- Relax the shoulders and open the chest.
- If the hips are shifting side to side the seat is incorrectly positioned.

Caution: Stop immediately if pain is felt on the pubic bone or in the knee joint.

Rowing machine

Stationary rowing is only suitable for postnatal women who had experience of this equipment before their pregnancy and have achieved a degree of postnatal abdominal stabilisation and strength. It is a very effective method of training, working both the upper and lower body, but requires a high level of motor skills to perform safely and effectively. The risk of leaning too far back makes this activity unsuitable for inexperienced rowers; weak abdominal muscles will be unable to maintain adequate support for the spine and doming may occur. It is also an intensive method of training that should be gently reintroduced to the experienced rower.

NB It is unlikely that this equipment will have been used during pregnancy due to the severely decreased range of movement caused by the bump!

Key points:
- Maintain correct neutral alignment and sit tall.
- Draw navel to spine throughout.
- Keep knees aligned – avoid rolling in.
- Draw the shoulder-blades down and keep the chest open.

- Avoid locking elbows or knees.
- Keeping the arms close to the body.
- Keep the back in an upright position – do not lean backwards.
- Do not slump forwards during the return phase.

Caution: Leaning back with weak abdominals may cause doming or back pain; do not allow the knees to hyperextend.

Stepping machines

The elliptical stepper is preferable to the basic stepper which carries greater risks than some of the other cardiovascular training methods. Stepping is a fully weight-bearing exercise of moderate impact demanding a high degree of pelvic movement. An effective workout requires full range of movement, but this may place too much stress on the sacroiliac and symphysis pubis as the pelvis rocks from side to side with each downward movement. Range of movement can be reduced by taking shallow steps which will help to maintain correct pelvic alignment, but this may be hard to sustain over a prolonged period of time and may still cause pressure on the sacroiliac joints. It may be necessary to hold on to the handrails to maintain correct upright posture if the weight of the breasts is pulling the body forwards. This supported position will reduce the effectiveness of the workout but may provide a welcome break. Pace should be moderate; speeding up may not give the knees sufficient time to extend or cause them to lock out. Local muscle fatigue will determine the duration of this activity. Many of these concerns are reduced with the elliptical stepper as the action is less stressful to the pelvis.

Key points:
- Maintain correct neutral alignment and stand tall.

- Draw navel to spine frequently.
- Avoid locking the knees out.
- Keep knees aligned – avoid rolling in.
- Relax the shoulders and open the chest.
- Keep the back lifted with a slight forwards lean – hold the handrails for support if required.
- Keep the head in line and avoid looking down at the feet.

Caution: Do not allow the knee joint to lock out; avoid excessive pelvic movement.

Cross-trainers

Co-ordinated use of the upper and lower body has greater cardiovascular benefits but requires core strength to prevent rotational movements occurring in the pelvis and torso. It is recommended that cross-training is postponed until core abdominal strength has been gained. Key points additional to those for the stepper:

- Hold the bars at elbow height.
- Keep the elbows as close to the body as possible.
- Draw the shoulder-blades down and allow a gentle forwards and backwards arm motion.
- Add intervals of increased upper body work.

Swimming

This is an excellent activity that can be commenced when bleeding and discharge has completely finished. The buoyancy of the water eliminates stress to the joints and pelvic floor and reduces the weight of the breasts. It also has additional relaxing qualities and, providing the water temperature is not too cold, can be very therapeutic. Swimming lengths of the pool is a most appropriate method of cardiovascular training that can be taken at a gentle or moderate pace. Breaststroke is the most leisurely stroke, although the spine may be at risk of hyperextension if the head is held too high out of the water. This stroke may also be unsuitable if pain has previously been experienced on the pubic bone, as the wide abduction and adduction of the legs may aggravate the condition. Front crawl and backstroke, however, require vigorous arm movements, which may encourage milk flow. The demanding, highly physical action of butterfly should be confined to the very fit, experienced swimmer. Further discussion can be found in Chapter 13.

Structure of a cardiovascular session

Warm-up

As with any exercise session, a comprehensive warm-up should be performed to prepare the body for exercise and prevent injury. The warm-up should include:

Mobilising movements which take the joints through their full range in a slow, controlled manner. This stimulates the production of synovial fluid found in the joints which acts as a lubricant, allowing smooth, easy movement. The mobilised joints should be relevant to the type of activity to follow and should include both the upper and lower body.

Pulse-raising activities to increase heart rate gradually. The cardiovascular system needs a gentle introduction to exercise to avoid sudden stress, therefore a period of low-intensity activity (40–60% MHR) is essential. Movements should be rhythmical and continuous and increase gradually in intensity. It is preferable for this preparatory phase to be specific to the main activity to be undertaken as

it also provides an opportunity to rehearse the movement patterns and increase co-ordination, i.e. use the bike to raise the pulse if it is to be used in the main workout.

Stretches for those muscle groups to be used in the proposed activity (*see* pages 97–100). These stretches should be held for approximately eight seconds; some will need support for balance. If using cardiovascular machines, some of these stretches can be performed whilst still on the equipment.

The duration of the warm-up should be approximately 10 minutes to allow sufficient time for all sections to be completed effectively.

Cardiovascular training

- Select the desired activity from the choices available, with particular consideration to their postnatal suitability.
- Consider intensity and duration based on fitness level, postnatal factors and the type of activity.
- Maintain strict adherence to the correct exercise technique throughout the workout.
- Draw navel to spine throughout the activity.

Cool-down

The cool-down session should include:

Pulse-lowering activities to decrease the intensity and lower the heart rate gradually. This period of approximately five minutes gives the heart rate time to readjust and allows time for the removal of waste products from the working muscles. Inadequate recovery time and early cessation of the activity could result in blood pooling in the legs causing dizziness and fainting. It is recommended that the heart rate drops to less than 100 bpm before stopping the activity to avoid this occurring. If the session has been undertaken on equipment, in particular a treadmill, it is important to pause for a minute or so on completion, before leaving the equipment to allow the feeling of continual motion to pass. Getting off the equipment too quickly may cause dizziness.

Stretches for all the muscle groups that have been worked (*see* Chapter 8). If equipment is used, some of the stretches could be performed while still in position – this would provide a longer recovery time and prevent the dizziness mentioned above. Seated and lying positions may be adopted providing the transition to the floor is taken with appropriate care for the abdominals. Stretches to maintain flexibility should be held in a static position for up to 15 seconds; the upper body positions will require slightly less time. Developmental stretching to increase flexibility is contra-indicated until joint stability has returned. Stretching is a very important part of the exercise programme and should never be omitted; in particular, the repetitive action of cardiovascular training may create muscle imbalance if stretching is not included.

Summary

- Regular cardiovascular exercise of the appropriate intensity, duration and type is beneficial to postnatal recovery and may assist weight loss.
- Low-impact activities are strongly recommended and correct joint alignment is essential.
- Increased Q angle will affect knee alignment.
- Dropped arches will affect foot strike during walking/jogging.
- High-impact activities will stress the joints, pelvic floor and breasts.
- Decreased joint stability increases the likelihood of ankle sprains.
- Navel to spine contractions are essential throughout all activities.
- Co-ordinated arm and leg actions require strong abdominal stabilisation.
- The breasts should be well supported with an appropriate sports bra.
- Vigorous arm work may cause the breasts to leak.
- Dehydration may reduce the amount of milk available for the next feed.
- Very intense training may give breast milk a sour taste.
- Training should build up to three sessions a week but should not exceed five.
- Intensity should be gentle to moderate during the early weeks (50–70% MHR).
- Ten minutes duration can gradually increase to 20–30 minutes depending on the intensity of the workout.
- Brisk walks with the baby can be integrated into the daily routine.
- Outdoor walking is particularly beneficial for assisting calcium absorption.
- Correct running style is essential to reduce risks.
- Recumbent bike is more suitable than the upright bike.
- Rowing is appropriate only for experienced participants who have regained a degree of abdominal core strength.
- An elliptical stepping action is preferable to the regular up and down movement.
- Swimming is an excellent cardiovascular activity.

RESISTANCE TRAINING

11

Benefits of resistance training

Increased strength and endurance, particularly in the upper body, is highly desirable, if not essential, postnatally and can be achieved much more effectively with the use of weights. The physical demands of lifting and carrying the baby and accompanying equipment suggest the need to develop upper body strength, and this cannot be fully achieved without the use of weights. A resistance programme that targets postural muscles, particularly those destabilised through pregnancy, and major muscles involved in lifting and carrying should be extremely beneficial in reducing the demands of everyday life. Additional benefits relate to increased muscle mass demanding greater energy expenditure and assisting with weight loss.

Implications

Joints and relaxin

Joint vulnerability is a key issue in the use of weights during the postnatal period and they should be introduced with caution to prevent injury. Correct posture and exercise technique is vital together with the selection of low-risk exercises. The symphysis pubis and sacroiliac joints need particular care and those muscles with attachments to the pelvis should be trained with caution. Movement of the symphysis pubis and sacroiliac joints during pregnancy and delivery may continue to cause problems postnatally (*see* Chapter 5). Symphysis pubis

pain is experienced around the area of the pubis, radiating into the groin and inner thigh. Strong resisted exercises for the adductor muscles, particularly with weights, are contra-indicated if pain is experienced in this area. Due to its attachment to the pubic bone, contraction of the adductor muscle may increase joint separation and lead to a chronic problem. Symphysis pubis and/or sacroiliac pain may also be experienced during abductor work particularly if correct pelvic alignment is not maintained.

Abdominal muscles

Resisted exercises for rectus abdominis and the obliques are contra-indicated until the former has shortened and realigned (*see* Chapter 2). TrA strengthening should be the priority and this can be achieved in a variety of ways as described in Chapter 2.

Level 1 rectus abdominis exercises (*see* page 30) can be undertaken alongside the TrA, but increased strength in the latter should be achieved before moving on to the gravity-resisted progressions of Level 2. Enormous gains can be achieved through the core training programme, which is far more relevant than utilising abdominal resistance equipment (*see* Chapter 8).

While the introduction of resistance equipment to train other muscle groups may be appropriate, reduced abdominal strength does raise concerns for postural alignment. If the core muscles are unable to stabilise the torso, spinal alignment may be compromised and injury occur. Overhead movements in particular, such as lat pull-down or shoulder press, need careful observation to ensure correct alignment is maintained – keeping the weights slightly forward and not lifting directly above the head will alleviate some of the risk. Rigorous performance of navel to spine contractions must be enforced with all exercises. The heavier the resistance the greater the workload on TrA to maintain stabilisation; progression should be dependent on the strength of the core as well as the prime mover.

Getting into and out of position should also be considered as the abdominal musculature can easily be stressed by poor transitions. Equipment that requires the participant to be in a supine position, e.g. bench press or recumbent leg press, should be avoided if doming occurs in the abdominals when moving into place (*see* page 28). The maintenance of neutral alignment is imperative in supine bench lying, and may be quite challenging to maintain while holding weights. Moving into and out of supine lying while holding the weights is contra-indicated at this stage.

Pelvic floor muscles

These muscles have stretched and weakened during pregnancy and may have been further stressed by a vaginal delivery (*see* Chapter 3). The pelvic floor, together with TrA, multifidus and diaphragm, form the core muscles that support and stabilise the spine and are activated together. If correct navel to spine engagement is undertaken, as discussed above, the pelvic floor will co-contract to lift and support the pelvic organs. Lifting heavy weights with poor core strength will increase the stress to these muscles as intra-abdominal pressure cannot be resisted and is forced downwards onto the pelvic floor. (*See* Chapter 8 for more details on core training.)

Breasts

A breastfeeding woman may have a reduced choice of equipment available to her. Selection of appropriate exercises should consider the increased size and the comfort of the breasts which will feel tender if squeezed or bumped. This will include any prone lying exercises, seated pec dec and all seated exercises with chest pads (preacher curl, triceps extension, seated row, etc.). Body positioning and joint alignment should not be compromised in order to perform such exercises comfortably; this particularly applies to prone lying, where placing the hands under the breasts to reduce the pressure may cause the spine to hyperextend. Free weights usage may necessitate slight adaptations to work within a comfortable range of movement, i.e. biceps curl adapted to hammer curl to avoid bumping the breasts with a bulky dumbbell. Consideration should also be given to the possible leakage of milk if an excessive amount of arm work is performed; body parts should be worked in rotation and repetitions closely monitored.

Carpal tunnel syndrome

Carpal tunnel syndrome is associated with oedema which compresses the nerves of the fingers as they pass through the narrow tunnel of bones in the wrist causing tingling and numbness in the fingers (*see* Chapter 5). This raises the following concerns for resistance training:

- Flexion of the supporting wrist joint during certain weight-bearing exercises (triceps kickbacks/single arm row) will further reduce blood flow to the fingers.
- Poor wrist/forearm alignment in any position may induce discomfort. Exercises using resistance bands need particularly close observation.
- Grip strength may be affected.

- Wrapping a resistance band around the fingers will further restrict blood flow.

Correct wrist alignment must be observed at all times, and although the gripped position of the fingers may still cause problems, over-gripping should be discouraged. Tingling or numbness is less likely to occur when the hands are in an elevated position as gravity is able to assist the draining of excess fluid.

Considerations

Strength or endurance?

Strength work should be avoided until the effects of increased relaxin on the body have ceased. This may take approximately five months or possibly longer if breast feeding. The increased elasticity of connective tissue in the muscles and joint attachments greatly increases the risk of joint injury when maximum load is used (*see* Chapter 1). Working to failure is likely to be detrimental to the joints and core stabilising muscles, which cannot withstand such high demands. This will compromise spinal safety and cause a rise in blood pressure through the induction of the valsalva manoeuvre (see below). Endurance work is strongly recommended, using a high rep range and low resistance.

What is the valsalva manoeuvre?

This is a condition associated with strength training, when pressure in the thoracic cavity increases through forced exhalation with the breath held. This can occur when a weight is too heavy or the muscles are fatiguing during the last repetition of a set. It causes a rise in blood pressure and increases intra-abdominal pressure, placing further stress on the abdominal and pelvic floor muscles.

Free weights versus fixed resistance equipment

Fixed resistance equipment cannot always replicate joint action and some of the positions may not be comfortable postnatally. Additionally, on some older equipment, where the range of movement is not adjustable, there is an increased risk of overextension, e.g. some pec dec machines – if the range is too large for the shoulder joint, hyperextension of the spine will occur. Another consideration is that the minimum resistance available on selected pieces of equipment may still be too heavy for some women.

Fixed resistance equipment does, however, provide a stable body position which is generally well supported. The pre-set range of movement previously mentioned can be advantageous, preventing overextension of joints, although range adjusters are now available with the majority of equipment. Much less skill is required to use fixed resistance equipment and it would seem to be a very appropriate method of training for an inexperienced person providing a comprehensive induction has been given.

Free weights, body bars and resistance bands are beneficial as they can replicate the action of the joint in a variety of body positions. They all, however, require body awareness and strong core stabilisation muscles to support the spine and prevent unnecessary movement. The heavier the resistance the greater the demand on the stabilising muscles and this should be considered when progressing exercises, even if the prime mover is coping adequately. The use of light equipment is recommended once a degree of core strength has been gained – close observation of technique is vital.

Position selection

Some fixed resistance equipment may be unsuitable due to body position. All seated exercises with chest pads (preacher curl, triceps extension, lever row) may feel extremely uncomfortable for women who are breastfeeding, as will prone positions, discussed earlier. The latter may also be inappropriate for women who delivered by caesarean section due to the possible discomfort experienced around the site of the scar. The supine position itself is appropriate but the transition into it may stress the abdominals and increase separation of the two muscular bands. Side lying, before rolling over onto the back, is strongly recommended for floorwork but is inappropriate on a bench as there is very little room for the manoeuvre. Many exercises using external resistance can be performed standing or sitting.

Range of movement

In order to work effectively, joints should be taken through their full range of movement, although particular care must be taken to prevent overextending, which will increase the risk of injury to vulnerable joints. The range of movement can be adjusted on some fixed resistance equipment and this may be necessary on the pec dec machine to prevent hyperextension of the spine. Range of movement can also be limited by double-pinning to maintain safety and comfort. On a total hip machine a safe range of movement is quite restricted for the gluteals and hamstrings unless the body alignment is taken forwards from the hips. Hyperextension of the spine will occur very early on in the movement if this is not observed.

How soon can training commence?

All participants, experienced or not, must increase their core strength before introducing weights. Following a satisfactory postnatal check-up, a programme of core training should be undertaken (*see* Chapter 8) and once this has developed the exercises should be rehearsed, without the resistance. This will train TrA to respond in that particular movement pattern before the weight is added. Particular emphasis should be placed on the core programme for experienced participants, who may wish to return to the gym immediately and recommence where they left off!

What are the intensity recommendations for experienced trainers?

Assuming the above has been adhered to, experienced trainers are advised to work at 70 per cent of the weight lifted prior to pregnancy. This may gradually increase, over a period of weeks, to the pre-pregnancy resistance, but the emphasis should remain on endurance training until joint stability has returned. As well as core strength, intensity considerations should also relate to breastfeeding as fatigue, dehydration and the production of lactic acid may affect milk availability and taste. Strength training should not resume until breastfeeding has ceased and joint stability returned.

What are the intensity recommendations for inexperienced trainers?

Again, assuming the above recommendations have been adhered to, newcomers to weights should begin with the lightest weight available. This practice run provides a better feel for the movement than the initial weight-free rehearsal and an opportunity to focus on the required technique. Once this has been achieved the intensity selected should be sufficient to induce mild fatigue on the last repetition of a 12–20 rep set. Correct breathing must be practised to avoid the risk of breath-holding and the consequential induction of the valsalva manoeuvre. Joint alignment and exercise technique is absolutely vital at this time. The newcomer needs careful guidance from an instructor on transitions into and out of machines, handling free weights, and the exercise itself. Close observation and correction is expected.

Target muscle groups

Abdominal and pelvic floor muscles have the highest priority, the former should not be trained with weights in the postnatal period (*see* Chapters 2 and 3) Other key muscles include those lengthened and weakened by pregnancy postural changes, i.e. gluteus maximus and trapezius/rhomboids, together with other muscles involved in lifting and carrying, i.e. pectorals, latissimus dorsi, biceps, triceps and quads. Weakened joint structures all need increased muscle mass to provide support, i.e. gluteus medius/minimus, adductor group, vastus medialis, lower trapezius, deltoids and rotator cuff.

Are there any exercises that should be avoided?

The adductor group muscles should be exercised with caution due to the vulnerability of symphysis pubis and its potential stress when the muscles are contracted. Exercises for the abductor muscles may also cause problems here or at the back of the pelvis in the sacroiliac joints. Exercise or transitory positions which

cause the abdominals to dome should be eliminated until appropriate recovery is made. Any exercise performed with incorrect technique should be stopped immediately. The suitability of the upright row should be considered in relation to target muscles and postnatal posture. Upper trapezius is already very tight and this exercise will accentuate tension in the area; breasts may also compromise correct alignment. Studio resistance training is discussed in Chapter 12.

Guidelines for a resistance training session

- Select appropriate exercises for the target muscle groups.
- Consider position and range of movement.
- Select an appropriate weight to experience mild fatigue on the last repetition.
- Assume correct starting position with good postural alignment and neutral spine.
- Maintain navel to spine contractions throughout the repetitions.
- Complete 12–20 repetitions in one set.
- Observe strict adherence to correct technique.
- Rest and repeat; the lift may be repeated immediately after a short break of approximately 45 seconds, or may be repeated later in the workout.
- Exercise body parts in rotation – one upper body exercise followed by one lower body exercise to prevent early fatigue.

Table 11.1 shows the postnatal concerns and additional teaching points relating to the more regularly used fixed resistance machines.

Table 11.1	Considerations in the use of fixed resistance machines	
Resistance Exercise	**Postnatal concerns**	**Additional specific teaching points**
Chest press	Weak TrA Locking elbows Wrist/forearm alignment Transition into position (if supine)	Maintain correct postural alignment Draw navel to spine throughout Slide shoulder-blades down Draw ribcage down Lengthen away from sit bones Seated option is preferable
Pec dec	Getting into position Unstable base (if stool) Range of movement Weak TrA Back hyperextension	Maintain correct postural alignment Draw navel to spine throughout Slide shoulder-blades down Draw ribcage down Elbows/wrists remain on pads Lengthen away from sit bones Keep both hip bones facing forward
Triceps push down	Breasts (if high pulley) Weak TrA Locking elbows Wrist/forearm alignment	Maintain correct postural alignment Draw navel to spine throughout Slide shoulder-blades down Draw ribcage down Lengthen away from sit bones Seated option is preferable
Shoulder press	Weak TrA Back hyperextension Locking elbows Unstable base (if stool)	Maintain correct postural alignment Draw navel to spine throughout Slide shoulder-blades down Draw ribcage down Lengthen away from sit bones Keep both hip bones facing forward
Lat pull-down	Symphysis pubis (if straddling bench) Weak TrA Back hyperextension Locking elbows Wrist/forearm alignment	Maintain correct postural alignment Draw navel to spine throughout Slide shoulder-blades down Draw ribcage down Lengthen away from sit bones Keep both hip bones facing forward

Seated cable
  row
	Sacroiliac joints (if
	   shuffling into position)
	Weak TrA
		Maintain correct postural alignment
		Draw navel to spine throughout
		Slide shoulder-blades down

Table 11.1	Considerations in the use of fixed resistance machines	
Resistance Exercise	Postnatal concerns	Additional specific teaching points
	Back hyperextension Doming abdominals Locking elbows Forward flexion	Draw ribcage down Lengthen away from sit bones Maintain upright stance throughout Seated option may be inappropriate if breastfeeding

Biceps curl	Breasts
	Range of movement
	Weak TrA
	Deadlifting the bar
	Locking elbows
	Back alignment
		Maintain correct postural alignment
		Draw navel to spine throughout
		Slide shoulder-blades down
		Draw ribcage down
		Lengthen away from sit bones
		Preacher curl unsuitable if breastfeeding.
		If bar on low pulley affects range of movement,
		    exchange for handle attachment and
		    perform one side at a time.

Leg press	Weak TrA Locking knees Doming abdominals Incorrect knee alignment	Maintain correct postural alignment Draw navel to spine throughout Slide shoulder-blades down Draw ribcage down Lengthen away from sit bones
Leg extension	Getting into position Pelvic care Weak TrA Doming abdominals Incorrect knee alignment Locking knees	Maintain correct postural alignment Draw navel to spine throughout Slide shoulder-blades down Draw ribcage down Lengthen away from sit bones Avoid swinging the leg

Leg curl	Getting into position
	Pelvic care
	Weak TrA
	Doming abdominals
	Incorrect knee alignment
	Locking knees
		Maintain correct postural alignment
		Draw navel to spine throughout
		Slide shoulder-blades down
		Draw ribcage down
		Lengthen away from sit bones
		Seated option preferable. Standing low pulley
		    with cuffed ankle needs back care. Avoid
		    prone lying bench version

Abductor press	Getting into position	Maintain correct postural alignment Draw navel to spine throughout

Table 11.1	Considerations in the use of fixed resistance machines	
Resistance Exercise	Postnatal concerns	Additional specific teaching points
	Sacroiliac and symphysis pubis cautions Weak TrA Back hyperextension	Slide shoulder-blades down Draw ribcage down Lengthen away from sit bones Adjust to suitable range Perform both legs together
Adductor press	Getting into position Symphysis pubis caution Weak TrA Back hyperextension	Maintain correct postural alignment Draw navel to spine throughout Slide shoulder-blades down Draw ribcage down Lengthen away from sit bones Adjust to suitable range Perform both legs together
Calf raise	Weak TrA Reduced ankle stability Incorrect knee alignment Incorrect weight placement	Maintain correct postural alignment Draw navel to spine throughout Slide shoulder-blades down Draw ribcage down Lengthen the spine Lift the arches of the feet

Selected exercises using portable resistance equipment

The following exercises are intended for use once some core stability has been gained. For variety, three types of resistance have been selected, i.e. bands, body bars and dumb-bells as these are the most readily available, practical pieces of equipment. Some of the exercises can be performed with all three, whilst others are only suitable for one type of resistance. To avoid repetition only one version is described but alternative equipment is offered when appropriate.

Bands

Rotator cuff

Purpose: to strengthen the muscles of the shoulder joint which have been affected by pregnancy postural changes. External rotation is more beneficial for kyphotic changes.

Preparation
Stand in correct posture, with feet hip-width apart and spine in neutral. Hold a resistance band in front at waist height with palms facing in, thumbs on top and wrists/forearms aligned. Band should be straight but not taut. Elbows should be drawn into waist, shoulders and ribcage drawn down.

Ex 11.1 Rotator cuff

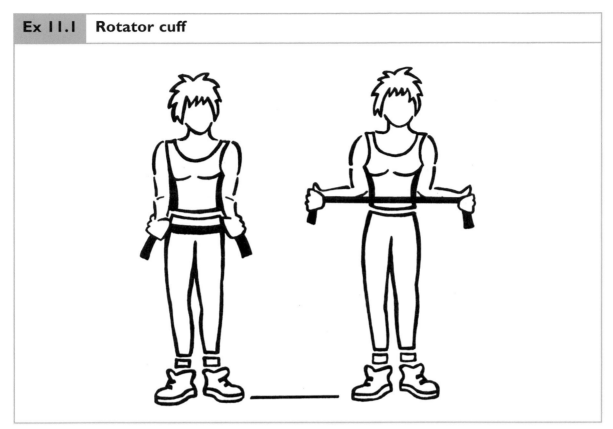

Action

Inhale to prepare, and as you exhale draw navel to spine and open forearms out to the side, pulling the resistance band outwards whilst keeping elbows tightly into waistline. Inhale to release and return with control.

Technique tips
- Ensure navel to spine contraction with each repetition.
- Maintain correct postural alignment throughout – do not lean back as the arms open.
- Use the abdominals to draw the ribcage down.
- Slide the shoulder-blades down as the arms open.
- Maintain wrist and forearm alignment.

Progression

Use a stronger resistance band to intensify the exercise.

Trapezius squeeze

Purpose: to strengthen the mid-trapezius and rhomboid muscles to reduce kyphotic changes.

Preparation

Stand in correct posture, with feet hip-width apart and spine in neutral. Hold a resistance band in front at chest height with thumbs together on top. Lift the elbows and keep wrists/forearms aligned. Shoulders and ribcage drawn down.

Ex 11.2 Trapezius squeeze

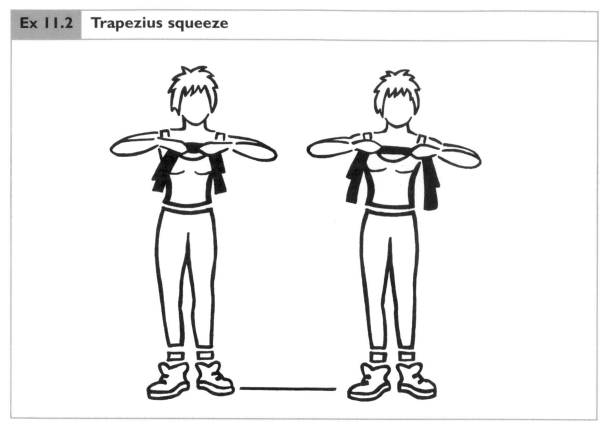

Action
Inhale to prepare, and as you exhale draw navel to spine and pull the band apart, drawing the shoulder-blades downwards and inwards. Inhale to release with control.

Technique tips
- Ensure navel to spine contraction with each repetition.
- Maintain correct postural alignment throughout – do not lean back as the arms open.
- Use the abdominals to draw the ribcage down.
- Maintain wrist and forearm alignment.
- Keep the elbows lifted.
- Draw the shoulder-blades down as the arms open.

Progression
Double the band up to increase the resistance before moving to a stronger band.

Seated row

Purpose: to strengthen the latissimus dorsi, trapezius and biceps to assist postural correction and lifting/carrying.

Preparation
Sit on the floor with legs extended in front, knees slightly bent. Ensure you are positioned on your sit bones – you may need to bend the knees a little more for comfort. Wrap a resistance band around the soles of the feet and hold each end with thumbs on top, arms reaching forward.

Ex 11.3 Seated row

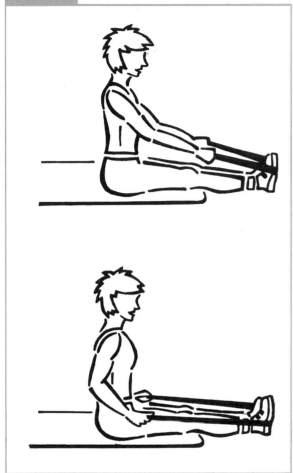

Action

Inhale to prepare, and as you exhale draw navel to spine and pull the arms back, leading with the elbows and bending them in close to the body. Keep the back in an upright position. Inhale to return to starting position, keeping the upper back lifted.

Technique tips

- Ensure navel to spine contraction with each repetition.
- Maintain   correct   postural   alignment

throughout: avoid arching the back as the arms draw back; avoid bending forward on return; keep lifted on your sit bones, don't rock back.

- Use the abdominals to draw the ribcage down.
- Keep the shoulder-blades drawing down throughout.
- Maintain wrist and forearm alignment.
- Keep the elbows close to the body.
- Bend the knees further if the hamstrings are pulling.

Progression

Use a stronger resistance band to intensify the exercise.

Pectoral press

Purpose: to strengthen the pectoral muscles to increase breast support and assist with lifting and carrying.

Preparation

Stand in correct posture, feet hip-width apart and spine in neutral. Wrap a resistance band around your back and under your armpits, and hold the ends with arms extended to the side at shoulder height. Soften your elbows, relax your shoulders and ensure wrists and forearms are aligned. Band should be straight and taut.

Action

Inhale to prepare, and as you exhale draw navel to spine and press the arms in front of the chest so that forearms cross. Keep the elbows slightly bent and shoulders down. Inhale to return to start position. Repeat, alternating the top arm.

Technique tips

- Ensure navel to spine contraction with each repetition.

Ex 11.4 | Pectoral press

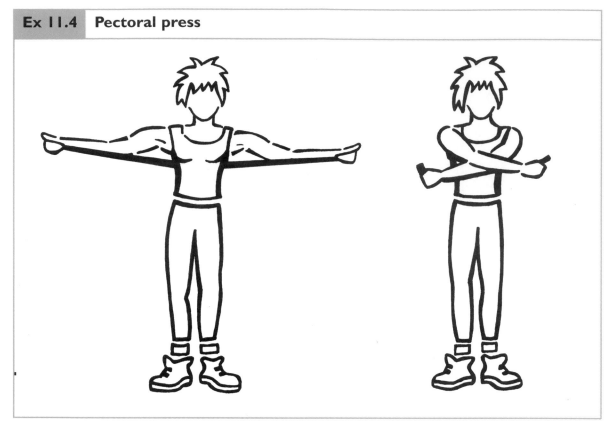

- Maintain correct postural alignment throughout.
- Keep the back lifted as the arms cross.
- Avoid hyperextending the spine as the arms open.
- Use the abdominals to draw the ribcage down.
- Keep the shoulder-blades drawing down throughout.
- Maintain wrist and forearm alignment.
- Aim to cross the elbows in front of the chest.

Alternative
This exercise can also be performed lying supine with dumb-bells or body bar lifting to the ceiling above chest.

Body bar

Biceps curl
Purpose: to strengthen the biceps muscles to assist with lifting and carrying.

Preparation
Stand in correct posture, feet slightly wider than hips with spine in neutral. Hold the bar with an underhand grip, arms shoulder-width apart. Extend the arms towards your thighs and draw the elbows into your sides, keeping wrists and forearms aligned. Slide the shoulder-blades down and soften the knees.

Ex 11.4 Bicep curl

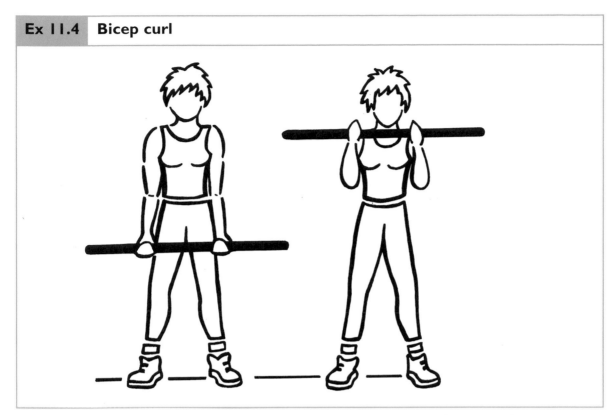

Action

Inhale to prepare, and as you exhale, draw navel to spine and curl the lower arms up towards the shoulder, keeping the spine in neutral. Inhale as you lower the arms with control, straightening the elbows but not allowing them to lock out. Maintain wrist/forearm alignment throughout.

Technique tips

- Ensure navel to spine contraction with each repetition.
- Stand tall, maintaining correct postural alignment throughout.
- Draw the ribcage down as the arms are raised to avoid leaning back.
- Avoid locking out the elbows as they lower.
- Keep the shoulder-blades drawing down throughout.
- Maintain wrist and forearm alignment.
- Perform slowly with control.

NB If this feels uncomfortable for large breasts use dumb-bells instead of a body bar and perform as hammer curl to avoid brushing the breasts.

Alternative

This exercise can be performed seated or kneeling, with an option to use dumb-bells instead. Alternatively, fix a resistance band under both feet, hip-width apart, or under one foot, in split stance, if the band is short. Hold around each end of the band with thumbs on top, forearms parallel to the floor. If this is too intense, work one arm at a time so the band is longer.

Ex 11.5 | Shoulder press

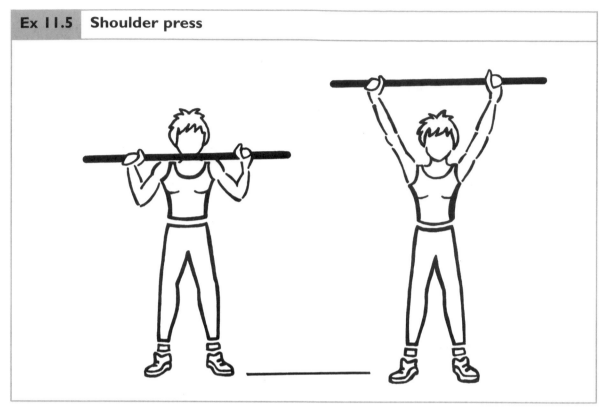

Shoulder press

Purpose: to strengthen the deltoids, triceps, pectorals and to assist with postural realignment and lifting and carrying.

Preparation
Stand in correct posture, feet slightly wider than hips with spine in neutral. Hold the bar in front with an overhand grip, arms shoulder-width and a half apart, at shoulder height, with elbows lifted and wrists/forearms aligned. Slide the shoulder-blades down and soften the knees.

Action
Inhale to prepare, and as you exhale draw navel to spine and press the bar upwards – straightening but not locking out the elbows and keeping the shoulder-blades down. Inhale to lower the arms to shoulder height with forearm fixed.

Technique tips
- Ensure navel to spine contraction with each repetition.
- Stand tall, maintaining correct postural alignment throughout.
- Keep the arms slightly forward to avoid arching the back.
- Draw the ribcage down as the arms are raised, to avoid leaning back.
- Avoid locking out the elbows as they straighten.
- Keep the shoulder-blades drawing down throughout.
- Maintain wrist and forearm alignment.
- Perform slowly with control.
- Practice without the bar first, to rehearse the

Ex 11.6 Standing squat

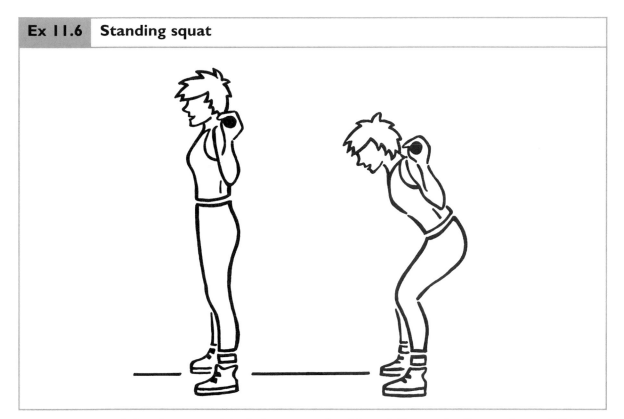

movement and develop correct technique.

Caution: Taking the bar behind the head may cause the spine to hyperextend.

Alternative
This exercise can also be performed seated or with dumb-bells.

Standing squat

Purpose: to strengthen the gluteals, hamstrings and quadriceps muscles to assist with postural realignment and lifting.

Preparation
Stand in correct posture, feet slightly wider than hips, with spine in neutral. Hold the bar across the shoulders with an overhand grip, arms shoulder-width apart, elbows down. Slide the shoulder-blades down and stand tall.

Action
Inhale to prepare, and as you exhale draw navel to spine and bend the knees, hingeing at the hips as you lower but maintaining neutral spine. Do not bend below 90 degrees. Inhale to return to the upright position without locking out the knees.

Technique tips
- Ensure navel to spine with each repetition.
- Maintain correct postural alignment throughout – do not lose the abdominal support.
- Take the body weight back towards the heels.
- The bar should move up and down in a straight line.

- As you lower, think of lengthening the spine away from the floor.
- Keep eye line ahead – avoid looking down.
- Keep knees aligned in parallel.
- Imagine you're lowering yourself onto a chair.
- Fully extend the knees and hips as you return
- Perform slowly with control.
- Practice without the bar first, to rehearse the movement and develop correct technique.

Caution: The back is greatly at risk with this exercise if the abdominals are not drawn in prior to movement.

Dumb-bells

Lateral raise

Purpose: to strengthen the deltoid muscles to assist with lifting and carrying.

Preparation
Stand in correct posture, feet slightly wider than hips with spine in neutral. Hold a dumb-bell in each hand and rest on the outside of the thighs with palms facing inwards. Tuck the thumbs around the dumb-bells to take a firm grip and soften the elbows. Slide the ribs and shoulder-blades down and soften the knees.

Action
Inhale to prepare and as you exhale, draw navel to spine and lift the arms up the side to shoulder height, rotating the arms as you lift so that the thumbs tilt downwards. Inhale to lower slowly, rotating the arms back to the starting position. Keep the shoulder-blades down, elbows slightly bent and wrist/forearms aligned.

Ex 11.7	**Lateral raise**

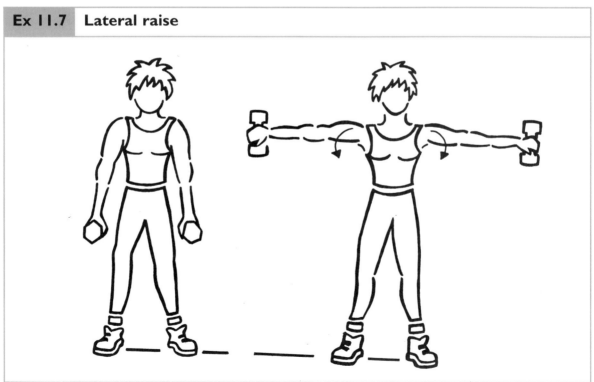

Technique tips
- Ensure navel to spine contraction with each repetition.
- Stand tall – maintaining correct postural alignment throughout.
- Curve the arms slightly forward to prevent the back hyperextending as they lift.
- Lengthen away from the shoulder joint as you lift and draw the shoulder-blades down.
- Lead with the knuckles and keep the elbows soft.
- Maintain wrist and forearm alignment.
- Perform slowly with control.
- Practice without the dumb-bells first, to rehearse the movement and develop correct technique.

Alternative
This exercise can also be performed with a resistance band under one or both feet, holding each end, with knuckles down. The length of the band will determine the range of movement possible.

Triceps kickback

Purpose: to strengthen the triceps muscles to assist with lifting and carrying.

Preparation
Kneel sideways on a chair with the left foot on the floor, knee soft, level with the lifted right knee. Rest the right hand on the chair in front of the knee, to form a triangular base with the legs, and lean forward. Hold a dumb-bell in the left hand, palm facing in, and bend the elbow, keeping the upper arm fixed into the side of the body. Tuck the thumbs around the dumb-bell to take a firm grip. Ensure the shoulders are square to the front and the spine is in neutral.

Action
Inhale to prepare and as you exhale, draw navel to spine and extend the forearm backwards, keeping the upper arm fixed into the body and wrist/forearm aligned. Inhale to bend the elbow and lower the forearm.

Ex 11.8	Triceps kickback

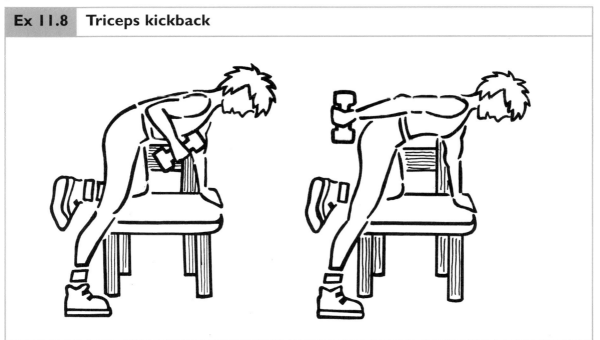

Technique tips
- Ensure spine is correctly aligned before commencing.
- Repeat navel to spine contraction with each repetition.
- Avoid twisting in the upper body.
- Keep the upper arm held into the body.
- Slide the shoulder-blades down.
- Maintain wrist and forearm alignment.
- Perform slowly with control.
- Practice without the dumb-bell first, to rehearse the movement and develop correct technique.

Alternative
This exercise can also be performed with a resistance band under the supporting hand. The length of the band will determine the range of movement and degree of resistance.

Single arm row

Purpose: to strengthen the latissimus dorsi, posterior deltoids, biceps and trapezius.

Preparation
Kneel sideways on a chair with the left foot on the floor, knee soft and level with the lifted right knee. Rest the right hand on the chair in front of the knee, to form a triangular base with the legs, and lean forward. Hold a dumb-bell in the left hand, palms facing in with elbow straight and dumb-bell reaching towards the floor. Shoulders square to the floor and spine in neutral alignment.

Action
Inhale to prepare and as you exhale, draw navel to spine and lift the dumb-bell up towards the armpit, keeping it close to the body. Inhale to lower down to the floor, maintaining neutral alignment and keeping the weight evenly distributed between the three points of support.

Technique tips
- Ensure spine is correctly aligned before commencing and throughout.
- Repeat navel to spine contraction with each repetition.

Ex 11.9	Single arm row

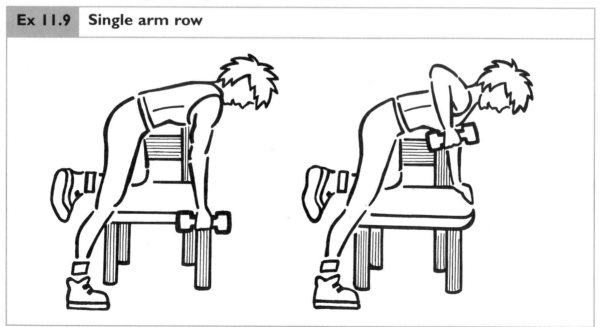

- Avoid twisting in the upper body.
- Keep the dumb-bell close to the body.
- Avoid locking out the elbow as the arm extends.
- Slide the shoulder-blades down.
- Maintain wrist and forearm alignment.
- Perform slowly with control.
- Practice without the dumb-bell first, to rehearse the movement and develop correct technique.

Alternative
This exercise can also be performed in the same position with a resistance band under the supporting foot, or standing in split stance with slight forward lean, band under the front foot, lifting both arms together. The length of the band will determine the range of movement and degree of resistance.

Dumb-bell lunge

Purpose: to strengthen the gluteals and quadriceps muscles to assist with bending and lifting.

Preparation
Stand in correct posture, feet hip-width apart and spine in neutral. Hold a dumb-bell in each hand and rest on the outside of the thighs with palms facing inwards. Tuck the thumbs around the dumb-bells to take a firm grip and soften the elbows. Take a large step forward with one foot, maintaining hip-width, and lift the back heel off the floor. Centre your weight between both legs and soften the knees.

Action
Inhale to prepare, and as you exhale draw navel to spine and bend both knees, lowering the back knee towards the floor. Keep the body weight centred to ensure correct knee

Ex 11.10	**Dumb-bell lunge**

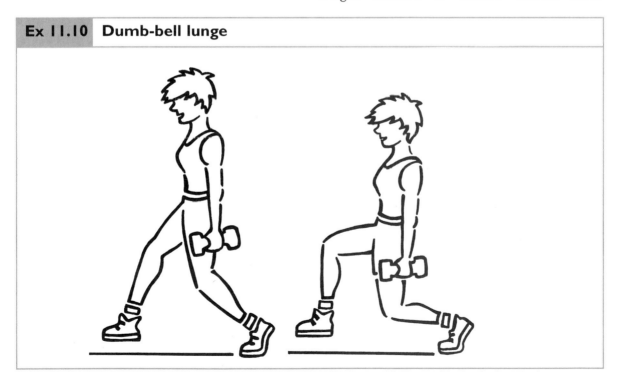

alignment. Inhale to return, to standing keeping the spine in neutral and the shoulders down. Repeat several times on one side before changing.

Technique tips
- Ensure navel to spine with each repetition.
- Maintain correct postural alignment throughout.
- Keep the front knee aligned over the ankle and back knee under the hip.
- Avoid locking out the knee on return to standing.
- Think of lengthening the spine away from the floor as you bend.
- Perform slowly with control.
- Practice without the dumb-bells first, to rehearse the movement and develop correct technique
- Keep the range of movement small initially and progress to the deeper bend when strength has been gained.

Caution: If pain or discomfort is felt in the knees, perform without the dumb-bells. This is an intensive exercise and should commence with low repetitions.

Alternative
This exercise can also be performed with a body bar held across the shoulders.

Summary

- Increased strength and endurance, particularly in the upper body, is extremely beneficial postnatally.
- Increased muscle mass assists with weight loss.
- Postural muscles should be targeted, particularly those destabilised through pregnancy, as well as the major muscles involved in lifting and carrying.

- The lingering effects of relaxin may increase the risk of injury when weights are involved. These may persist for longer if breastfeeding continues.
- Working to failure is contra-indicated until joint stability has returned. It also places tremendous stress on the weakened pelvic floor muscles, particularly if the valsalva manoeuvre is used.
- Hyperextension of any joint should be avoided.
- Correct posture and exercise technique is vital.
- Core stabilisation is essential. It is inappropriate to introduce weights until TrA strength has increased.
- Resistance equipment for the abdominal muscles is inappropriate at this stage.
- A safe transition to the supine position should prevent doming of the abdominal muscles.
- Breastfeeding reduces the choices of suitable, comfortable equipment.
- Range of movement may need to be reduced to maintain comfort and safety.
- Carpal tunnel syndrome may affect the use of some equipment.
- Fixed resistance equipment provides stable positions but works within a pre-set range of movement.
- Portable resistance equipment can replicate joint movement more effectively but requires strong core muscles to stabilise.
- Experienced trainers are advised to work at 70 per cent of the weight used prior to pregnancy; inexperienced trainers to mild fatigue on the last repetition of a 12–20 rep set.

GROUP EXERCISE SESSIONS

12

This chapter looks at different types of classes and discusses their suitability for postnatal women and the main considerations for participation.

Specific postnatal exercise class

Suitability

This is the most suitable method of group exercise following a postnatal check-up. While this type of class will probably attract the less-fit mum who has not previously exercised, the serious exerciser may seek the additional and valuable social benefits of a specific postnatal class. A specialist class such as this will be valuable to all new mothers, regardless of the length of time that has passed since delivery; it is certainly suitable within the first year, and in fact the low-level, carefully structured programme is an excellent introduction to exercise at any time.

Considerations

Postnatal exercise sessions consider all the implications of pregnancy and delivery and the continuing effects of relaxin on the body. Movements are simple and easy to follow and floorwork concentrates on those muscle groups weakened as a result of pregnancy and delivery. A great deal of emphasis is placed on retraining TrA and pelvic floor and correcting poor postural alignment. All exercises are suitable and provision is made for alternative positions and/or exercises where appropriate.

The social and emotional benefits of a specific postnatal exercise session are invaluable. It provides an opportunity to meet other new mums and to offer support to each other over the concerns and anxieties frequently experienced with a new baby. It is also a non-threatening exercise environment with the majority of women concerned about the lack of muscular tone in their abdomen and their struggle to lose extra weight gained during pregnancy.

Pilates

Suitability

Pilates is ideal for postnatal women. It focuses on all the key areas affected by pregnancy and helps improve posture and increase core strength. The calm, controlled nature of pilates reduces the risk of joint stress, encourages correct alignment and aids relaxation and focus. The benefits are highly appropriate:

- Flattens abdominals and restores natural posture
- Isolates, activates and conditions deep muscles
- Develops strength, flexibility and endurance
- Builds core abdominal and back strength
- Tones and elongates without adding bulk
- Alleviates pain and tension
- Increases circulation

Most of the exercises in the abdominal and core stability chapters of this book are Pilates-based.

Considerations

It is strongly recommended that women inexperienced in Pilates commence with a beginners' course to learn the essential principles. Even experienced participants would benefit from returning to basics for a short while. It takes time to co-ordinate breath and movement and correct sequencing is the essence of the technique. Attending a general class with no prior knowledge or with incorrect sequencing from forgotten technique will stress the abdominal musculature and may strain the back.

Prone positions may be uncomfortable for breastfeeding women and adaptations may be necessary. If performed, back extension work should be approached with caution to ensure the abdominals are engaged prior to lifting. Exercises involving rectus abdominis may be inappropriate if the muscles still have separation or may stress the neck due to increased tension or incorrect alignment. Commencement of gravity-resisted exercises for the obliques should be delayed until TrA strength has been regained and rectus abdominis shortened and strengthened.

Yoga

Suitability

Yoga is an excellent activity for postnatal women providing pregnancy and postnatal changes are considered. The benefits are highly appropriate:

- Relaxes and rejuvenates the body
- Aids digestion and helps resolve constipation
- Promotes circulation
- Releases muscular tensions
- Improves balance
- Increases body awareness

Many styles of yoga are now taught, some are more suitable for postnatal women than others. All styles are descendants of the original **Hatha** yoga, which encompasses mind, body and spirit. It is the easiest, most relaxing of styles and is the most suitable for postnatal women. **Ivengar** is stricter than Hatha and involves holding poses for longer, which may be too demanding for postnatal women. **Ashtanga** is an advanced form, performed faster than the others, which links postures together into a series of movements. It requires strength, stamina and flexibility. It is unsuitable for postnatal women.

Considerations

The main concerns relate to range of movement and joint alignment. Pushing the body beyond its natural range is contra-indicated at this time and it is expected that postnatal participants will be closely observed and modifications offered wherever appropriate.

Movements, such as the cobra, which encourage lumbar hyperextension, need modification to prevent further stress to the spine and abdominals. Pelvic rotational movements may stress the sacroiliac joints and wide standing postures may cause discomfort to the symphysis pubis. Changes in femur alignment may trigger knee and pelvic discomfort in warrior pose, although this posture is particularly good for stretching tight hip flexors. Downward-facing dog is excellent for lengthening spinal extensors, performed with heels up and knees bent, although the breasts may drag uncomfortably in this position. Inversions should be avoided in the early weeks and reintroduced with modifications, i.e. wall-supported shoulder stand. This position is beneficial for aiding venous return and reducing swelling, and can be very helpful for re-educating the pelvic floor muscles.

Stretch class

Suitability

The gentle, seemingly undemanding style of a stretch class is often preferred to an energetic, lively workout. Stretching can be extremely beneficial in reducing muscle tension, and will help to improve poor posture often adopted as a result of pregnancy and continuous babycare. The calm, controlled nature of a stretch class may also help to reduce emotional stress and encourage the body to rest and relax.

Considerations

While stretching has valuable benefits, flexibility work should be avoided in the early months after delivery as this may result in overstretching of the ligaments supporting the joints. A ligament that is overstretched at this time may not retract to its original length, leaving the joint vulnerable to injury. Stretching to maintain mobility/flexibility is strongly recommended. Joint alignment should be considered in all stretch positions to ensure safety is not compromised. Adductor stretches should be avoided if pain is experienced on the pubic bone as this may indicate increased movement in the symphysis pubis joint.

Some seated floor positions may be uncomfortable for the perineum, and prone lying will obviously be unsuitable if breastfeeding. Stretches for the abdominal muscles are inappropriate at this time since the emphasis of postnatal abdominal recovery is on shortening and realigning the muscles. Those who had a caesarean delivery may experience discomfort with stretches that pull on the abdomen, e.g. gluteal stretch and lying body stretch.

Body conditioning class

Suitability

This is an umbrella term for a variety of class types, e.g. legs, bums and tums, body sculpt, etc. It is a popular choice postnatally as it has no cardiovascular component and includes a large proportion of muscular endurance work for the major muscle groups, abdominals included. (Many postnatal women avoid classes that might include any type of jumping because of discomfort to the breasts and the risk of leaking due to the weak pelvic floor.)

Considerations

As always joint alignment and range of movement are important considerations to avoid stress to the joints, but they are particularly crucial if hand weights or body bars are used. Overextension of the elbows, knees or spine may occur as the muscles fatigue, therefore it is important to select light weights and, if necessary, perform fewer repetitions. Although many of the exercises may be performed on the floor, the pelvis should still be treated with the greatest respect. Pain or discomfort may be experienced around the symphysis pubis or sacroiliac joints whilst performing specific exercises or during transitions. Exercises for the abductors and/or adductors may be particularly problematic. Abdominal work should focus on TrA and progress according to the guidelines given in Chapter 2. The temptation to return to fast, vigorous abdominal work should be avoided as it will be counter-productive.

Prone floor positions will probably be

uncomfortable if breastfeeding. Some of the exercises can be adapted to a box position on elbows and knees while others will need alternative exercises. Seated floor positions may be uncomfortable for the perineum and may also require a change of position.

High/low aerobic classes

Suitability

High-impact aerobics is unsuitable because of the increased stress to the joints, breasts and pelvic floor. Low-impact moves are much safer and can be equally effective. When the pace of an aerobic session increases and the music becomes more motivating there is a danger that momentum may cause joint misalignment, particularly if participants are not familiar with the movements.

Considerations

Movements that stress the joints do not necessarily involve jumping; some seemingly low-impact moves can still create an increased degree of stress purely through poor performance. Marching on the spot, for example, if performed with a heavy downward stamp, can create a similar amount of force to that of jumping. Keeping the body lifted and emphasising the upward movement will reduce the impact considerably. Fast knee-bending movements increase the impact on the pelvic floor and may feel most uncomfortable. Such movements should be performed at half speed or an alternative exercise provided. Correct joint alignment should be closely monitored and particular care taken to avoid excessive pelvic movement. The symphysis pubis should be protected by reducing the width of sidesteps and the sacroiliac joints kept in line by ensuring

movements on one leg maintain a lift through the supporting hip.

Upright posture is also extremely important, particularly when arm movements increase. There may be a tendency to lean too far forward when the arms are used in front of the body, particularly if the breasts are heavy. This places additional strain on the thoracic spine and encourages round shoulders. When the arms are taken behind the body or above the head the back may hyperextend and increase stress to the lumbar spine. Reducing the range of backward arm movements and keeping the arms further forwards when working above the head will help to maintain correct spinal alignment, providing the abdominals remain tightly pulled in.

Excessive use of wide-range arm movements, particularly with momentum, may cause the breasts to leak. Exercise intensity should be kept to a moderate level – working too hard will cause fatigue and may affect milk quality and quantity. Supportive footwear is essential to provide adequate shock absorption and increased ankle stability. A supportive bra is also essential to reduce the movement of the breasts and minimise bounce.

Dance-based workouts

Suitability

This is an umbrella term for an enormous variety of styles – some more appropriate than others for postnatal women. Most comprise fun, motivating routines to improve co-ordination, agility and cardiovascular fitness and burn unwanted calories – generally, without unduly taxing the body.

Considerations

Participation in the postnatal period needs caution if excessive pelvic movements, found in many dance styles, are performed. Continuous pelvic gyration may stress unstable pelvic joints that are recovering from pregnancy changes. Once again music and atmosphere are the greatest cause of concern as the mood takes over. Breasts may need additional support for this type of activity.

Step class

Suitability

This cardiovascular activity can be a valuable form of exercise if undertaken at an appropriate level. If the combinations are simple and easy to follow, step may be a far more beneficial workout for the inexperienced exerciser than attempting to follow the co-ordinated movements of an aerobics class. There are concerns, however, relating to the continuous, repetitive nature of the activity as well as the speed and complexity of some classes, particularly for a newcomer. All these factors place additional stress on the joints, still lacking stability from the continuing effects of relaxin, particularly if alignment and technique are weak. The intensity and complexity of the class together with the ability of the instructor to provide alternative exercises is most significant in determining suitability for attendance.

Considerations

The stepping action should be reviewed to ensure the whole foot is placed on the step every time and the ankles braced to prevent them rolling over. When stepping up, the knees should straighten but not lock out and the pelvis remain in a neutral position. The spine is particularly vulnerable, especially when lifting the leg behind when there is a natural tendency to arch the back; upper body weight should be adjusted forwards and the abdominals held in tightly to prevent this occurring. Step height must be considered in relation to the degree of pelvic rocking from side to side; excessive movement will stress the sacroiliac and symphysis pubis joints and should be avoided. Side leg raises may cause twisting in the pelvic joints. The ballistic nature of power moves may also cause additional stress to the joints and pelvic floor. The breasts need appropriate support to minimise movement and bounce and may feel very uncomfortable if power moves are attempted. Correct upper body posture must be maintained throughout with particular reminders to keep the back extended and draw navel to spine.

If the stepping part of a step class continues for more than 40 minutes the session may become too demanding, in which case regular blocks of active rest should be incorporated into the combinations to reduce the intensity and provide short breaks. This could simply be marching or sidestepping on the floor, temporarily excluding the arm work. Continuing at a higher intensity will not only cause muscular fatigue, but concentration and co-ordination may decrease, which could lead to joint injury. Additionally, fatigue, dehydration and lactic acid may affect milk quality and milk production. Excessive use of the arms may cause the breasts to leak.

Studio cycling

Suitability

This is an intense cardiovascular and muscular endurance workout set to music. Although the intensity is self-regulated the motivating nature of the workout encourages participants to maintain the group pace, which may push a postnatal woman to work too hard, too soon. This has implications on breastfeeding and energy levels. Additionally, the saddle of the bike may be extremely uncomfortable for the perineum and the forward leaning position may cause a high degree of distress to the pubis. Studio cycling can only be recommended after individuals have returned to a reasonable level of fitness through other, more suitable training methods.

Considerations

Although a variety of riding positions may be adopted during a session, the forward stance emphasises the kyphotic posture which a postnatal woman is probably trying to correct. An upright riding posture should be encouraged whenever possible, and all positions must activate core stabilisation. As with regular cycling, the seated position on the bike is crucial to prevent unnecessary pelvic movement and avoid stress to the knees. A comfortable seat height should allow the knees to extend but not lock out, and the pelvis should remain still. Care should be taken with sprinting as the momentum of the spin can easily wrench the knees out of alignment if concentration is momentarily lost. Joints continue to be at risk as long as breastfeeding continues.

Studio resistance

Suitability

As a general rule, high repetition, low resistance weight training is a recommended activity for postnatal women (*see* Chapter 11), however, in a studio environment, it may not be as appropriate. While it encourages correct lifting technique and increases muscular endurance, its performance to music raises concerns. Studio resistance training is certainly *unsuitable* for women returning to exercise for the first time after delivery.

Considerations

Music is a performance enhancer and, when combined with a light resistance, presents additional risks for postnatal women. Music sets the pace of the session, adds momentum and dictates the number of repetitions and speed of performance. Relaxin-affected joints need additional protection when a weight is introduced and technique is of paramount importance. Varied use of speed provides contrast and dynamics but faster movements may encourage joint overextension or result in poor technique. Even with the lightest resistance, a five-minute sequence that focuses on one muscle group may cause early fatigue and loss of technique.

Poor core strength is another area of concern as there will be insufficient stability for the spine (*see* Chapter 8). Strong centre control is essential to prevent injury and must be developed before commencing this type of training. Weak, stretched abdominals are particularly at risk when getting into and out of the supine bench positions. Holding the barbell to do this places enormous additional stress on the abdominal muscles and puts the back at risk. Doming may occur during this transition.

Increased size of breasts may reduce the range of movement and change body alignment during 'the clean'.

Postnatal women wishing to participate in studio resistance training should take the following steps:

- Improve core strength with TrA exercises (*see* Chapter 2) or by participation in a specific

postnatal exercise programme.
- Rehearse the movements without weights to programme TrA activation into each movement pattern.
- Use the lightest resistance available.
- Perform *all* repetitions slowly.
- Maintain good joint alignment throughout.
- The instructor should assist by passing/taking the barbell during the supine lying section.

Studio martial arts

Suitability

This is a powerful, dynamic workout, performed to music, and is inappropriate for postnatal women until at least six months after delivery. Its explosive, athletic style requires a large degree of core strength to maintain good postural alignment whilst the rapid, jabbing-type movements may compromise joint safety by increasing the risk of overextension or misalignment. Although range and speed of movements can be self-monitored, music and group atmosphere are likely to encourage increased effort over and above the desired postnatal level.

Considerations

Experienced participants may return to this style of activity, once core strength has been regained and breastfeeding ceased. The following areas need consideration:

- Rotational hip movements with kick (particularly for women who experienced sacroiliac problems)
- Knee-snapping actions
- Wide or deep lunges – particularly if symphysis pubis problems previously existed

- Fast forearm jabs
- Postural alignment
- Abdominal support

Summary

- A specific postnatal exercise class is strongly recommended for all levels of fitness. In addition to appropriate structure and content it offers other important social benefits.
- Pilates is strongly recommended.
- Hatha yoga is extremely therapeutic providing postnatal changes are considered and modifications taught.
- Stretch classes are beneficial in reducing muscle tension providing developmental stretching is avoided.
- Body conditioning workouts should consider intensity and body positioning.
- High-impact aerobic movements are unsuitable – low-impact movements are more appropriate but joint and pelvic care is necessary.
- Dance-based workouts need caution where excessive pelvic movements are involved.
- Step training of the appropriate intensity may be valuable although repetitive joint action should be considered.
- Studio cycling is unsuitable until a degree of cardiovascular fitness has been gained.
- Studio resistance sessions are unsuitable until core strength is developed.
- Studio martial arts are unsuitable until relaxin effects have been withdrawn from the body and core strength developed.

WATER WORKOUTS

13

Postnatal benefits of water workouts

- **Reduced joint stress**
  One of the major benefits of water workouts is the reduction in the amount of stress to weight-bearing joints. Structures that have been destabilised during pregnancy through the effects of relaxin and increased weight gain, are supported by the water when submerged.
- **Increased circulation**
  The pressure of water exerted on the blood vessels stimulates the circulation and increases stroke volume. This induces a lower working heart rate than on land. Improved circulation also helps resolve constipation.
- **Increased venous return**
  Water pressure encourages a more effective return of blood and prevents blood pooling in the legs. This is helpful for improving the condition of varicose veins.
- **Increased urinary output**
  Increased circulation improves blood flow to the kidneys which increases urinary output. This helps with the loss of excess fluid retained during pregnancy.
- **Reduced swelling**
  Water pressure forces retained fluids out of the swelling into the circulation. This is particularly helpful for pelvic floor repair.
- **Reduced muscle soreness**
  Exercising in water predominantly consists of concentric muscular work (this principle changes when flotation equipment is used). Muscular soreness is generally produced by eccentric work, therefore the after-effects of a water workout are felt less than on land.
- **Soothing and calming effects**
  Water can be very therapeutic in aiding postnatal recovery. The slower actions of the body and the massaging effects of the water induce a feeling of composure and relaxation. This often continues after the workout has finished.

Implications

Joints

Effects of gravity on the body are reduced by 80 per cent when submerged at chest depth. This cushioning of the body allows the joints a greater range of movement but water resistance slows movements down and reduces the risk of injury from this greater range of movement. Immersion to the waist reduces the effects of gravity by only 50 per cent; this has implications on joint and breast stress when jumping or if large-range upper body movements are performed.

Abdominals

TrA plays a key role in trunk stabilisation (*see* Chapter 2). In water the workload intensifies, and the deeper the water the greater the workload. As the body becomes more buoyant, TrA must stabilise the torso to allow the arms and legs to move and prevent the body moving in the opposite direction. In group sessions the workload intensifies with increased turbulence. This repetitive postural training is an excellent method of recovery for the abdominals but should be performed in shallow water initially to avoid overworking. Movements that require strong rotation of the trunk should not be performed if the abdominals have a separation of more than two fingers. With the resistance of the water this may encourage further separation as the oblique muscles pull on rectus abdominis (*see* Chapter 2).

Pelvic floor

Due to the buoyancy of the body in water, risk to the pelvic floor is significantly reduced. Reduced gravitational pull makes it easier to engage the pelvic floor muscles, so if an individual is experiencing difficulty with this exercise on land it may be a good alternative. The pressure of the water on the perineum will help to reduce any lingering swelling around the episiotomy or tear site by dispersing retained fluids and speeding up the healing process. Increased urinary output, in water, fills the bladder more quickly and it is usually necessary to urinate more frequently.

Breasts

Breasts must be supported during exercise of any type to prevent sagging and overstretching. Many swimsuits do not have the additional support of a shelf bra sewn into the garment; this could result in heavy breasts being supported by just one layer of very stretched fabric. It may be necessary to wear a bra under the swimsuit to reduce bounce. If the breasts remain immersed under the water there is much less risk of damage, but if the water level is below the breasts the delicate breast tissue is just as vulnerable as during land-based exercise. Even with appropriate support, the drag effect of the water on the breasts when jumping can be extremely uncomfortable.

When exercising in waist-deep water it is strongly recommended to adopt a wide leg base and bend the knees; not only does this keep the breasts immersed but it also provides greater stability and a more effective workout for the arms.

Feeding before exercising is always recommended (if baby is obliging) but this may not prevent a loss of milk if vigorous large-range arm work is continued. Exercising in very warm water may encourage milk flow. Breast milk is unlikely to be affected by intense activity, as it is on land. This is due to the lower heart rate response experienced in water and the more effective use of the aerobic energy system resulting in reduced production of lactic acid.

Considerations

Water resistance

The resistance of water is 12 times greater than that of air, and when the body is immersed the resistance is present in all directions of movement. Group exercise sessions create turbulence, which further increases water resistance and can make it a very demanding activity. The intensity of the workload is determined by the amount of effort used – the greater the effort, the higher the workload. Speed increases the intensity to three times the level of that on land so fast movements cannot be continued for very long but can be interspersed between slow sections. The interval method of training is particularly useful when returning to exercise, as the more demanding sections can be of short duration in the initial sessions with the majority of the workout pitched at a gentle to moderate intensity.

Pool temperature

The temperature of the water is very significant, the high 80s (°F) being the ideal temperature providing the workout is not too intense. Warmer water increases the elastic qualities of the muscles and help to loosen the body, but it may also encourage milk flow from the breasts. Exercising in water that is too hot may cause the body to overheat and dehydrate. Water that is too cool may constrict blood vessels as the circulation is diverted away from the skin to maintain core temperature. This increases energy expenditure but may reduce transport and consumption of oxygen (Lawrence 1998).

Pool depth

The depth of the pool is relevant to both safety and effectiveness of exercise. Working out in chest-high water will support the joints, breasts and pelvic floor and significantly reduce the risk of injury and discomfort to these structures. It will also ensure a more effective workout than waist-high water by providing increased resistance to the upper body if the arms remain immersed. If positioned in waist-high water it is recommended to adopt a wide base and bend the knees in order to keep the breasts underwater.

When can you start?

Gentle swimming can be commenced when vaginal discharge has completely finished - this may vary between three and five weeks after the birth. Other, more vigorous, water-based activities may commence following a satisfactory postnatal check-up.

Shallow water workout

Suitability

A shallow water workout is undertaken in water that is chest-high or less. This is a popular activity, performed to music, and is similar to a land-based exercise to music class, performed at a slower speed.

Considerations

Exercising in an appropriate depth of water is crucial to joint safety, breast comfort and exercise effectiveness. Whilst chest-high water is preferable, a workout can be safely and effectively undertaken in waist-high water if a wide leg base is adopted and the knees remain bent. Jumping or springing movements should be included only if the breasts remain supported by the water and even then the drag of the water on the breasts may be uncomfortable. Strong rotational movements with the torso immersed should be avoided if the abdominal muscles remain separated. Exercising in a group increases the turbulence of the water and adds a greater resistance to the workload. TrA has to work much harder to stabilise the body and strong limb movements are needed to maintain balance. Equipment such as webbed gloves, floats, buoys or bands may be used in a shallow-water workout to increase the resistance.

Deep water workout

Suitability

Deep water workouts are not suitable for postnatal women. Due to the major role of TrA needed to stabilise the spine, participation should be postponed until abdominal strength has been regained. The weak abdominal musculature will be unable to maintain correct alignment and recovery may be jeopardised. Deep water is ideal for relaxation with the use of buoyancy aids.

Swimming

Suitability

Swimming is an excellent postnatal activity. It provides cardiovascular as well as local muscular benefits. Moderately paced swimming over a prolonged period of time will also utilise additional calories and help with weight loss. Gentle swimming can be particularly relaxing; the rhythmic action of the stroke, the feeling of weightlessness and the soft muffled sounds created by the water provide a calm, therapeutic quality not found in other activities.

Considerations

Despite the supporting effects of the water, any stroke performed with the head lifted too high out of the water will increase compression of the cervical spine. This position causes the hips to sink and increases lumbar lordosis. Swimming in a head down-position, realigns posture and allows the body to move more quickly through the water. Breaststroke leg action should be avoided if pain is experienced in the symphysis pubis as the wide abduction and adduction of the legs may aggravate the condition.

Summary

- Water workouts are particularly beneficial to postnatal women for joint and circulatory reasons.
- Stress to weight-bearing joints is greatly reduced.

- Body weight is reduced by 80 per cent when immersed to the chest.
- Body weight is reduced by 50 per cent when immersed to the waist.
- Water pressure stimulates the circulation and improves several postnatal conditions.
- TrA muscles work hard to stabilise the spine in the water.
- Exercising the pelvic floor in water is particularly helpful for muscular rehabilitation.
- Adequate breast support is essential.
- The breasts are at risk if they are not immersed – the knees should be bent to lower the body if exercising in waist-deep water.
- The drag effect of the breasts through the water when performing jumping movements may be very uncomfortable.
- Breast milk is unlikely to be affected by the intensity of water workouts.
- Gentle swimming can commence as soon as discharge has ceased; more vigorous workouts should wait until after the postnatal check.
- Water workouts can be very demanding if the resistance of the water is used correctly.
- Deep water workouts require strong abdominal muscles to maintain spinal stability.
- Swimming provides excellent cardiovascular and local muscular benefits.
- Hyperextension of the cervical and lumbar spine may occur if the head is held too high out of the water.

RELAXATION

14

In addition to regular exercise, rest and relaxation should be an essential part of a new mum's lifestyle.

Why is relaxation so important?

The arrival of a new baby places enormous physical and emotional demands on a woman, and unless adequate time is given to recharge her batteries she may experience mounting tension and fatigue, which could lead to stress.

What is stress?

Stress is a threat to the body, either in the form of real danger, which requires immediate and fast reactions, or as a result of a series of problems and pressures that build up over a period of time. The body responds to stress by making various changes to prepare for the impending 'conflict'. Unfortunately we are unable to distinguish between real danger and emotional pressure, so if the situation or threat does not require a physical response, such as running away from danger, the body has no way of dispersing it. The continual presence of stressful situations demands the muscles to be in a state of constant 'readiness' which is exhausting for the body.

Postnatal stress factors

Everyone is subjected to the stresses of everyday life, but a new baby brings additional physical and emotional pressures.

Physical factors may include:
- fatigue due to lack of sleep;
- sore, heavy breasts;
- sore perineum;
- constipation;
- pain or aching in the joints.

Emotional factors may include:
- being unable to settle baby;
- baby crying for long periods;
- concerns about the amount of feed baby is taking;
- having no time to do anything;
- unable to fit into normal clothes;
- feelings of loss of independence;
- feelings of inadequacy.

What happens to the body under stress?

The body becomes aroused and this is reflected outwardly by postural changes:

- head and body bent forwards;
- shoulders elevated;
- elbows bent and close to the body;
- fists clenched;
- legs crossed and ankle flexed (if seated);
- jaw tightly shut and teeth clenched.

Other, more complex changes may occur inside the body. The heart rate, blood pressure and breathing rate increase, blood is diverted away from the skin and digestive system to the lungs and skeletal muscles ready for action, the mouth becomes dry and sweating increases.

Once the situation has been dealt with, the body will return to normal with no harm done. If pressures continue, however, and the body is subjected to prolonged periods of arousal, strain will begin to show, resulting in tension, frustration and fatigue.

Coping with stress

The first stage of dealing with stress is recognition of the condition. Pressures build up slowly, one on top of the other and the body forgets how it feels to be calm and at ease. If the cause can be identified, the problems will be easier to deal with. Postnatal women may need reminding of their limitations, and be able to admit when they feel they can't cope.

Time out and relaxation

Taking time out is essential, and although she may feel it is inappropriate and self-indulgent, a woman should try to take the opportunity as often as possible. Her partner will probably enjoy the opportunity of spending time with the baby without her watchful eye; and although copious instructions will be left, he will probably manage very well! Taking up offers of assistance from others should be encouraged, as long as mum understands that things may be done differently. Concerns over this may increase her feelings of anxiety rather than making her pleased that the job has been done. Time off does not necessarily mean leaving the house; an allotted period of time at home, to spend as she chooses, may be an appropriate alternative. A period of relaxation is recommended.

Methods of relaxation

There are various methods of relaxation – the following three tend to be the most commonly used.

- **Contrast method**. This requires the individual contraction and release of all large muscle groups throughout the body. This method may not, however, provide sufficient opportunity for the tense muscle to release; if the muscle is already feeling tense and tight it is unable to let go and remains in a slightly contracted state.
- **Visualisation or imagery**. This involves the selection of a pleasant image that stimulates happy thoughts and feelings, but as this is mental imagery the physical state of the muscles is unaffected. There is also the possibility that an image may induce feelings of tension if bad experiences are visualised.
- **Physiological relaxation** (also known as the Mitchell Method). This method is widely taught during the antenatal period and, due to its simple, exact technique, is the most appropriate to continue into the postnatal period and beyond. It is based on the principle of muscles working in pairs – a muscle must relax to allow the opposing muscle to contract. The procedure and sequence of this method is explained on the following page.

When is the best time for relaxation?

Whenever an appropriate opportunity arises! Setting time aside after a feed, when baby may sleep for a while, or alternatively if baby feeds well, it may be appropriate to attempt a short period of relaxation whilst he is on the breast, assuming there are no other children around to keep an eye on or who may interrupt. Although this may not be as effective as relaxing alone, a comfortable, well-supported position will allow some degree of relaxation. Having learnt the skill of relaxation the body is able to let go much quicker. This means utilising more opportunities to switch off for five minutes at appropriate times during the day.

Where is the best place to relax?

Wherever a comfortable position can be adopted. Sitting at a table with head in hands, lying on the floor or bed, or sitting up in a comfortable, supportive chair. A cushion or pillow can be placed under the head to support the neck, or under the thighs if lying down to make the back feel more comfortable.

Preparing to relax

It is important to wear warm, comfortable clothing without restriction. Cushions and pillows can be used to support as necessary and a blanket positioned nearby if required. Allow the body to sink into the support as you release yourself into position.

The Mitchell Method of relaxation

- Move each joint into a position opposite to that of stress, i.e. stretch the muscle which is causing tension.
- Stop the movement.
- Momentarily pause and consider how the new position feels. This gives the nerves time to register the change and makes it easier for the body to recall the position of ease again.

Relaxation sequence

The Mitchell Method recommends that each joint is taken through the procedure in a fixed order, as follows. The instructions are an individual variation on the original language stated by Mitchell.

1 Arms

Shoulders
- pull your shoulders down away from your ears
- stop pulling
- feel that your shoulders are lower and the neck longer.

Elbows
- move your elbows away from your body
- stop moving
- feel your elbows open and away from your body.

Hands
- stretch out your fingers and thumbs
- stop stretching
- feel your hands, fingers and thumbs fully supported; be aware of the surface underneath your fingertips.

2 Legs

Hips
- roll your hips outwards
- stop rolling
- feel your legs slightly apart and rolled outwards.

Knees
- move your knees into a comfortable position
- stop moving
- be aware of the new position of your knees.

Feet
- flex the feet, drawing your toes towards your face
- stop flexing
- feel your feet hanging loosely from the ankles.

3 Body
- press your body into the support

4 Head – press your head into the pillow/support
– stop pressing
– feel your head well supported by the pillow.

5 Face
Jaw – keeping your lips together, pull down your jaw
– stop pulling
– feel your teeth separated and your lips gently touching each other.

Tongue – move your tongue to the middle of your mouth
– stop moving
– feel the tip of your tongue touching your lower teeth.

Eyes – close your eyes (if not already closed)
– be aware of the darkness.

Forehead – raise your eyebrows towards your hairline
– stop moving
– feel your skin smoothing out and your hair moving.

6 Breathing – take a deep breath in (in your own time)
– feel the ribs moving outwards
– breathe out easily (in your own time).

– stop pressing
– feel the pressure of your body on the support.

Once the sequence has been completed it can be repeated again a little faster, after which you should remain in your relaxed position for as long as circumstances permit. The pleasant feeling of comfort you experience throughout your body is relaxation.

Waking up

When the relaxation is over:

- Remain in position and open your eyes.
- Consider your body positioning for a few seconds.
- Slowly rotate your wrists and then your ankles.
- Reach your arms up above your head and release.
- Reach your legs away from you and release.
- Reach arms and legs together and release.
- Bend your knees up, one at a time and place the feet flat on the floor.
- Roll carefully on to your side and rest there for a moment.
- When you feel ready to get up, slowly push yourself up with your hands and move into a sitting position.
- If time permits, remain in a comfortable seated position and perform the following remobilising moves.

Shoulder rolls

- Slowly circle one shoulder round in a large exaggerated way (forwards, up, back, down).
- Draw navel gently to spine and keep the rest of the body still.
- Repeat eight times on each side.

Neck mobility

- Sit tall and lengthen the spine.
- Draw the shoulder-blades down.
- Slowly take the head over to one side.
- Pause before returning to the upright position.
- Repeat on the other side.

Side bends

- Bend slowly to the side, resting the hand on the floor for support.
- Return to the central position and draw navel to spine.
- Repeat several times to alternate sides.

Spine mobility

- Round the back and slowly bring the shoulders and arms around in front at chest height.
- Lift and lengthen the body as the arms open to the side, drawing the shoulder-blades down.
- Feel the chest opening and the spine lengthening.
- Keep the abdominals lightly drawn in to prevent the back from arching.

Upward reach

- Place one hand on the floor beside the hip.
- Lift up through the body and reach the other arm up to the ceiling.
- Keep the body weight slightly forwards and the abdominals lightly drawn in.
- Lengthen through the side of the body.
- Lower the arm, keeping the body lifted and tall.
- Repeat on the other side.

To stand up

Ensure the transition to standing is performed safely. Keep the abdominals drawn lightly in and avoid twisting the back whilst moving onto the side, knees and feet together where possible. Avoid pushing firmly on to the front thigh to get up; use the strength of the legs to lift up to standing (*see* Appendix for full details).

Time constraints of full relaxation

If time and circumstances do not permit such a comprehensive relaxation on every occasion, this technique can be adapted for quicker use. The shortened version is ideal for use during a five-minute break in a comfortable chair.

Shortened version

Take the body through the same sequence, but use the end position of each body part as the only movement – this must be done slowly to allow time for the appropriate responses to occur. If the full relaxation technique is practised regularly you should find that your body easily adopts the new positions.

Summary

- Relaxation is necessary to counteract the effects of stress.
- Physical and emotional factors increases muscular tension.
- Stress becomes exhausting for the body over a period of time.
- Time out and relaxation is essential for new mums.
- Women should be encouraged to be honest with themselves and admit when they can't cope.
- Take every opportunity to switch off for five minutes.
- Teach the body how to relax.

TEACHING STRATEGIES

PART THREE

3

PLANNING A POSTNATAL EXERCISE SESSION

15

Venue

The ideal venue should be easy to reach by public transport, with adequate car parking space close by. Pushchair accessibility is important with sufficient standing room within the exercise area, or other allocated storage space. Heating, lighting, ventilation, toilets, telephone and all obvious necessities should, of course, be provided. The facility should be clean and spacious (appropriate to the number of participants), free from obstacles and with a non-slip floor surface. Mats are essential for the floorwork sections.

Promotion

Contact with health professionals

The health visitor at the local clinic is an essential link with the postnatal community. She is the principal healthcare professional involved with new mums from day 10 after delivery (the midwife may still be involved if there have been particular problems). The health visitor makes home visits to new mums and is responsible for the baby clinic at the local health centre/GP surgery. Close liaison between the exercise instructor and health visitor could be extremely beneficial in increasing the advice available to postnatal women and creating an interest in specific postnatal exercise sessions. Through this source it may also be possible to visit postnatal groups, by appointment, to recommend and demonstrate appropriate exercises and back care. This is an excellent method of professional promotion but may have to be undertaken on a voluntary basis.

Leaflets and posters

These can be placed in a variety of locations: surgeries, clinics, mother and toddler groups, playgroups, schools and sports centres, subject to the relevant approval.

Advertising

The NCT (National Childbirth Trust) is a very active organisation with branches all over the country. It is run predominantly by mums for mums and is an extremely successful network of support and advice for both ante- and postnatal women. For a small fee, advertisements can be placed in branch newsletters which are sent out quarterly to all members (branch details and contact numbers are available at the local library). Advertisements can also be placed in other non-specific newspapers, newsletters, journals, etc. The Baby Directory is a national publication, available to purchase from leading bookstores. The Parents Directory currently offers only North and South London publications and is distributed free through clinics, surgeries, and libraries (*see* Useful Contacts for more information).

Listings

Inclusion on the database listings provided by a library is another useful source of promotion. The library is an obvious public resource and the database holds information regarding class type, venue, day, time, contact number, etc. Some local authorities publish an information book detailing facilities available for the under-fives in the area; activities for parents are also listed.

Session organisation

Drop-in sessions can of course be helpful for postnatal recovery but effective progression can realistically be achieved only by organising the sessions on a course basis (approx. 6–10 weeks in duration). Women can then begin together on week one and undergo a gentle introduction to exercise in a controlled and organised way. Sessions can progress in intensity and duration with new exercises gradually introduced and practised, thus reducing the risk factors associated with irregular attendance.

An advance booking system is recommended to avoid the difficulties of individuals just turning up for a session; this method ensures that all participants have been screened and follow-up enquiries made if necessary. Pre-payment encourages the commitment of regular attendance and improves results. This system requires a certain amount of administration to be successful.

Screening

Screening is essential to clarify suitability and identify specific contra-indications or concerns. A postnatal screening form should establish the following:

- Date of delivery
- Type of delivery (vaginal/caesarian)
- Completion of postnatal check-up
- Result of postnatal check-up
- Type of feeding

- Joint or back problems
- Any other postnatal concerns
- Medical history
- Current medication
- Exercise history

Do babies come along too?

Babies generally accompany mums to postnatal exercise sessions and may be cared for in a crèche or remain in the practical area. A crèche allows mums a much-needed opportunity to be able to focus on themselves and work towards recovering their physical fitness. However, running a crèche is an involved and costly procedure and if it operates for more than two hours in one day it must comply with the requirements of The Childrens Act (1989), which also specifies that babies must have completed their full course of immunisations before attending. Operating a crèche for less than two hours has no statutory legal requirements but it is imperative that the facility provider ensures adequate provision is made for the care and safety of the children – participants who are unhappy about the standard of childcare will not return to the exercise session. Successful operation involves the employment of sufficient staff to care for a number of small babies; ensuring the room temperature remains warm and constant; and a registration system to identify babies with mums (and feeds if appropriate). Baby-changing and milk-warming facilities are useful but not essential. Adequate insurance cover must be taken out by the provider to cover the employees as well as the children.

If a crèche is not available, the class can still be extremely beneficial, if a little noisy at times! Babies are often content to sit in their car seats or bouncy chairs during the more active sections of the class and can join their mums on an adjacent mat during the floorwork. Changing the order of the aerobic and muscular strength and endurance components may help to entertain babies who become unsettled towards the end of the session – a flexible plan is essential with a group of unpredictable small babies! Although they may not achieve such a thorough or effective workout, women should be encouraged to come along with their babies rather than not attend – any exercise is better than none, and some sessions will be more successful than others. Most women are pleasantly surprised at the amount they can achieve.

Exercising with baby

Aerobic section

Carrying baby in a sling or just holding him is not recommended for this section. It is potentially dangerous for both mother and baby and should not be permitted. To maintain cardiovascular activity, it is recommended to push baby briskly up and down the hall in the pushchair. Unfortunately this may not be helpful in settling him as the pace may be too fast to induce sleep!

Floorwork

This is the time when baby is most likely to become unsettled. Exercising on hands/elbows and knees can work well with baby positioned on the floor in front of and between the hands. During press-ups, having baby positioned there not only keeps mum's body weight forward but it also encourages her to bend a little lower towards the baby, who often enjoys grabbing handfuls of her hair!

When supine lying, baby can adopt a variety of positions depending which part of the body is moving. Lying across mum's abdomen is probably the most practical position but he will need to be held there. This becomes more difficult when the legs are lifted to table top. Sitting baby up on the abdomen is not appropriate until he has head control as it is difficult to support him properly. He can easily tip forwards or slip sideways and this becomes distracting for the maintenance of mum's exercise technique. This position is much more appropriate once he can support his head himself, although mum may not enjoy him pushing his heels into her breasts! Using the baby as a resistance for upper body work is not appropriate until he has full head control. This is not recommended in a group situation.

Side lying positions are practical and comfortable for both mother and baby. Most floor stretches have seated alternatives when baby can be positioned seated in between mum's legs supported by her hands, if not required by the stretch, or by her knees in crossed leg sitting.

Structure and content

A postnatal exercise session is structured to incorporate all the components of fitness. The following structure is applicable to both an exercise to music or circuit environment.

Warm-up

To include warming, loosening and pulse-raising activities followed by simple static stretches.

Considerations
- Revision of static and dynamic posture, taking into account the changes which have taken place in the body since delivery
- Controlled use of full range of movement during mobility

- Moderately-paced pulse-raising activities
- Stretches, some with support, for muscles tightened during pregnancy (hip flexors, pectorals, etc.), as well as those to be worked during the session.

Aerobic component

This should include a gradual rise in intensity, a short maintenance period and a gradual decline in intensity. Initially this should be a shallow curve which becomes more defined as the course continues. Duration of the aerobic component may commence at approximately eight minutes and increase to 15–18 minutes over a 10-week period. There is insufficient time in a 60-minute class to do much more than this if adequate time is to be spent on the floorwork. The purpose of the aerobic component should be explained and its benefits clearly defined, as some women will be interested in the floorwork exercises only to flatten their abdomens.

Considerations
- Use simple and easy to follow moves.
- Keep to low-impact activity.
- Perform sufficient repetitions to enable achievement.
- Keep the intensity low to moderate (60–70 per cent max heart rate).
- Incorporate intermittent use of upper body work.
- Avoid fast knee-bending movements.
- Take care with long levers and momentum.
- Use standing circuit stations to avoid participants having to manoeuvre to the floor and up again at speed.

On completion of the aerobic component, if floorwork is to follow, supported standing stretches may be included for major muscle groups, in particular the legs.

Muscular strength and endurance component

This should include muscle groups:

- weakened by the effects of pregnancy (abdominals, pelvic floor lower trapezius and gluteus maximus);
- needed for lifting, carrying and caring for the baby (biceps, triceps, pectorals, quads, etc.);
- providing support for weakened joint structure (abductors, adductors, quads etc.).

Considerations
- Safe practice of getting down to the floor
- Controlled and appropriate transitions
- Comfortable positions for breasts and pelvic floor
- Alternative positions and/or exercises provided where appropriate
- Appropriate and effective pace
- Sensitive but effective use of sets and repetitions
- Controlled use of full range of movement where possible

If undertaken as a circuit this component should be taught as a command circuit, where all participants perform the same exercise. This provides a much more controlled environment when transitions, joint alignment and technique can be more effectively monitored. A multi-station circuit is inappropriate until all participants are familiar with all the moves. Observation is crucial.

The cool-down component

This should include stretches for all the muscle groups worked, a period of relaxation and a gentle wake-up.

Considerations
- Perform maintenance stretches only – no developmental stretches.

- Offer appropriate, comfortable positions for the individual.
- Provide alternative positions where appropriate, e.g. gluteal stretch and lying body reach for caesarian deliveries; some seated positions for those with a sore perineum may be uncomfortable.
- Comfortable stretches may be held for longer than eight seconds providing the range is not increased.
- Include a relaxation period. This is an essential part of the session and may be the only opportunity in the day for a new mum to rest and relax. There may not always be time to teach a full relaxation section, particularly towards the end of the course when the content is greater, but the opportunity to rest the body for a few minutes with the inclusion of a few key relaxation points will still be beneficial.

Progression

The following ideas for progression are suggested for a 6–10 week course:

Warm-up

The mobility and pulse-raising elements of the warm-up may remain exactly the same from week to week. If the participants are new to exercise it may take a few sessions to become familiar with the movements and to perform them correctly. Progression in this section is noticeable by a more effective performance of these movements. Combining the mobility and pulse-raising sections and introducing more co-ordination may reduce the quality of the work. Leg stretches could be progressed by performing them unsupported, assuming correct technique has been achieved. Upper body stretches are more appropriate to remain in isolation, although this will depend on motor skills.

Aerobic component

Increasing the duration of this section is the primary method of progression. Commence with about eight minutes of aerobic work at the beginning of the course and increase to about 15–18 minutes by the end, maintaining a moderate intensity. Movements should remain uncomplicated and easy to follow, as familiarity will improve performance and increase effectiveness. The curve of intensity may become more defined towards the end of the course, with a peak of slightly more intense activity in the middle of the component, although this would need to be carefully monitored. Depending on the ability of the group the pace may increase slightly and arm work continue for longer than in earlier weeks. To cater for unsettled babies it may be necessary to do two shorter aerobic sessions, with floorwork sandwiched between; planning for this is essential to avoid sudden changes from standing to floor and up again.

Muscular strength and endurance

The length of time spent on this section should stay the same or may need to decrease slightly if more aerobic work is included. However, more effective use of this time by quicker organisation and transitions and less rest allows additional exercises to be included and more sets to be performed. Exercise intensity can also be increased by performing more repetitions, reducing the speed of the exercise or altering the body positioning to increase the resistance.

Towards the end of the course, when several muscle groups have already been introduced and need to be worked, there may be a tendency to rush this component in order to complete them all. Whilst progression is important, the safe, correct performance of all exercises is essential and may result in some exercises, already taught, being omitted.

Cool-down

Comfortable stretches should remain the same throughout the course and alternatives found for those that are uncomfortable. Although only maintenance stretches are included, some of the more passive positions could be held for slightly longer providing no attempt is made to increase the range of movement.

It may be appropriate, as the course progresses, to extend the length of the relaxation as participants feel more able to relax and switch off. This will be dependent on whether babies are present and the total time available.

Due to the time constraints, instructors must be highly selective in their planning to enable progression to occur in all areas.

Summary

- The health visitor is the essential link with the postnatal community.
- Screening is an essential part of professional care.
- A course of fixed duration and organised attendance is recommended.
- Successful classes can be held with babies in the room.
- Floorwork adaptations may be necessary to accommodate baby.
- The structure and content of the session should consider the effects of pregnancy and delivery.
- Progression in all components of the session will help to improve physical fitness.

TEACHING AND EVALUATING A POSTNATAL EXERCISE SESSION

16

Essential specialist teaching skills

To teach this specialist group safely and effectively an instructor should be competent in the following areas.

Teaching points

Teaching points are essential for both the safety and effectiveness of exercise.

A range of teaching points should be used to ensure movements are performed in a safe and appropriate way. These should be relevant to the technique of each exercise/movement with particular concern for joint alignment and the maintenance of correct posture. Reinforcement of the essential points must continue for the duration of the session and be reiterated on each meeting. Teaching points should be delivered as short, clear statements focusing on the positive, preventative care necessary to avoid a problem occurring. Recurring points may be given in a variety of ways to maintain interest. When new exercises are introduced, teaching points should be delivered one at a time, continuing only when the previous one has been achieved.

Initially these teaching points will be concerned predominantly with the safety of the movements, but as the skill and awareness of the participants develop, so the focus should change to increase the effectiveness of each movement. It is vital that the use of these valuable points is accompanied by correct technical performance by the instructor.

Teaching position

The instructor should be positioned so that he/she can see, and be seen by, all participants in the group. This may involve a variety of changes during different sections of the session.

- Turning the whole group around to face a different direction gives participants at the back an opportunity to see. It also allows the instructor to view individuals previously positioned behind others.
- Moving in the opposite direction to the group during a circle activity provides the opportunity for individual eye contact. Stepping out of the circle or circuit allows the instructor to scan the whole group.
- Demonstrating movements from different angles highlights particular areas of concern, e.g. turning the body sideways to reinforce spinal alignment.
- Leading a set of exercises with the back turned to the group may be helpful if the mirrored version is confusing to the participants. A brief demonstration in this position should be followed by the instructor turning to face the group so that group performance can be observed in the usual way.
- Moving amongst the group whilst they continue the movement/exercise provides an opportunity to observe the specific technique of individuals from a variety of angles.

The successful use of a variety of teaching positions is solely dependent on the initial organisation of the group. If, due to lack of instructions, the participants face different directions, the position of the instructor will not be appropriate to everyone – this is particularly relevant during the floorwork.

Demonstration

Excellent personal performance by the instructor is essential. The demonstration of correct technique, good postural alignment, and clear, precise movements conveys very strong visual messages which, when combined with the appropriate verbal information, provide the participant with all the necessary tools for correct performance. Movements should be strong, deliberate and large to motivate and encourage the use of effort; this is particularly relevant to upper body movements which often become weak and unclear.

Explanations

Instructions for group organisation and explanations of new exercises should be delivered clearly and precisely. It is also helpful to explain the purpose of the exercises selected; if participants are aware of why they are doing them they will be more interested in the resulting benefits. Information should also be given as to where certain exercises should be felt; as well as consolidating correct performance, this method also draws the instructor's attention to individuals who are not experiencing sensation in the relevant area. The explanation for testing the abdominal muscles for separation, although quite complex, should be relayed in user-friendly terms so the participants can understand and experience the condition of the muscles for themselves. The pelvic floor also needs detailed explanation.

Voice

The voice should be clear and audible throughout the session, and delivered at an appropriate pace to enable participants to process the information and react accordingly. Tone, volume and mood should be varied according to the component being taught. Tone and volume may also change as the participants become more able; a gentle, persuasive approach to the initial sessions may develop to a much more dynamic, motivating style as the course progresses. Sensitivity and encouragement must be shown at all stages of a postnatal course.

Observation

Good observation skills are vital, predominantly for safety reasons. The ability to look at the performance of the group and pick out individual problems is an essential and invaluable skill, and involves close scrutiny of posture and joint alignment, particularly when speed and intensity increase. This may be extremely difficult to observe if movements continually change, so it is helpful when planning a session to ensure combinations are repeated sufficiently to allow effective observation. In addition to the technical criteria to be met, observation should also include eye contact with individuals. This projects concern for the individual herself, not only the body being moved, and helps to build confidence and rapport. It also encourages a more effective performance. Indications of fatigue and strain can be seen in facial expressions as well as the satisfied smiles of enjoyment and achievement.

Technically correct but ineffective performance requires a higher level of skill to recognise, but it is another vital element to successful teaching. Once participants become familiar with the content of the session their performance must be carefully monitored for the degree of effort used. Appropriate feedback is then required.

Feedback

There are three types of feedback:

- correction of inappropriate technique, speed or intensity;
- improvement of ineffective performance;
- praise and encouragement.

Poor technique must be corrected immediately to prevent damage to the vulnerable joints and muscles. Depending on the severity of the problem it may be necessary to make immediate eye contact whilst offering the correction to ensure the individual is aware of the level of concern. This can be reinforced if the teaching position is changed and the correct method demonstrated, highlighting alignment from a different angle. If this does not have the desired effect, it may be necessary to move alongside or immediately in front of the individual. Correct technique should then be reinforced every time this movement occurs during the session and should be reiterated in following weeks.

Giving feedback to improve performance is essential if exercise is to be beneficial. A lack of appropriate feedback often results in little effort being used, and although the moves are performed safely they are ineffective. The instructor must work hard to ensure individuals are putting sufficient effort into the movements and extending, bending, pushing, and pulling in the biggest, safest way. A more dynamic use of voice and body language is often very helpful. Fully extending the arms, pulling up through the legs as the knees straighten, and drawing the shoulder-blades down and back as the arms lower are all teaching points that

should help to enhance performance.

Praise and encouragement are essential in this rather technically oriented session. Positive feedback to participants will motivate, encourage better performance and, above all, increase self-confidence which may be lacking at this time.

Adaptations and alternatives

These may be necessary for the following reasons:

- discomfort experienced in the required position/movement;
- tiredness;
- inappropriate intensity.

A range of levels should be demonstrated in all components, whenever possible, so that participants can choose the appropriate level for themselves for that day. A varied selection of arm work during the aerobic component and a varied choice of body positions for press-ups, for example, are both relevant general alternatives which are offered to everyone. Specific adaptations for individual conditions should, where possible, involve the same muscle group, although if a similar body position is required it may still be inappropriate. If the position itself is causing the problem, an alternative exercise may need to be given in another position; navel to spine contractions or pelvic floor exercises are an ideal choice as they can be performed in any position.

Once again, if the session is to be effective, the level of intensity selected by individuals should be appropriate to their ability; very often the easiest option will be taken by individuals who can obviously cope with more. It is up to the instructor to educate the group about effective exercise and encourage awareness of full performance as often as possible. There will be occasions, often due to tiredness, when this degree of effort is not possible and should be dealt with sensitively.

Session evaluation

Evaluation plays a crucial role in professional development, yet unfortunately it is often a neglected part of teaching. Reflecting on a session previously taught will allow the instructor to identify areas for improvement. The following questions provide an idea of the depth of information necessary to make a comprehensive evaluation.

Structure and content

Safe structure

- Did you warm and loosen the body before stretching?
- Did you gradually increase the intensity of the aerobic work?
- Did you gradually decrease the intensity of the aerobic work?
- Did you stretch all the muscles which had been worked?
- Did you allow adequate recovery time?
- How can you improve this?

Safe content

- Did you consider joint alignment in all movements/exercises?
- Did you consider the degree of impact and stress to vulnerable areas (pelvis, abdominal and pelvic floor muscles, breasts)?
- Did you consider speed/pace and use of momentum?
- Did you include easy-to-follow movements?
- How can you improve this?

Effective structure

- Did you provide an effective warm-up?
- Did you incorporate all the components of fitness?
- Did you provide an effective cool-down?

Effective content

- Was the body effectively prepared for the exercise to follow?
- Was the exercise at an appropriate level?
- Was the aerobic component of sufficient duration? Could the participants have coped with more?
- Was the aerobic component of the appropriate intensity? Could the participants have coped with more?
- Did the floorwork target appropriate muscle groups?
- Did the floorwork include sufficient sets and repetitions? Could the participants have coped with more?
- Did you stretch out all the muscles which had been worked?
- Could the participants have used more effort in any areas of the session?
- How can you improve this?

Enjoyment

- Did you look at the faces of the participants?
- Did they appear to be enjoying the session?
- Did you ask them for feedback?
- Did you get any feedback from them?
- Did you enjoy teaching?
- How can you improve this?

Teaching

Teaching points

- Were the teaching points appropriate to the content?
- Did they highlight posture and exercise safety?
- Were there sufficient points given?
- Were they reinforced?
- Did you use a variety of terms to say the same thing?
- Were they delivered at an appropriate pace?
- Were they clear and to the point?
- Were they effective?
- How can you improve this?

Teaching position

- Did you vary your position to see all participants?
- Did you vary it to emphasise postural alignment?
- Did you vary it to demonstrate movements?
- Did you vary it to observe performance?
- How can you improve this?

Demonstration

- Did you perform with correct alignment?
- Did you demonstrate in a strong, dynamic way?
- Did you perform too much of the session?
- How can you improve this?

Explanations

- Were you clear and precise?
- Did you explain the purpose of exercises?
- Did you tell the participants where the exercise should be felt?
- Did you feel you were able to educate your group?
- How can you improve this?

Voice

- Were you clear and audible?
- Did you deliver at an appropriate pace?
- Did you vary your tone and volume according to the components?
- Did you show sensitivity?
- Did you motivate and encourage?
- How can you improve this?

Observation

- Did you observe incorrect technique?
- Did you observe ineffective performance?
- Did you make eye contact?
- Did you observe facial expressions?

Feedback

- Did you correct inappropriate technique?
- Did you reinforce teaching points?
- Did you improve ineffective performance?
- Did you encourage more effort from everyone?
- Did you encourage more effort from individuals?
- Did you praise good performance?

Adaptations and alternatives

- Did you offer a range of levels?
- Did you demonstrate all options?
- Did you offer alternative positions?
- Did you teach the alternative positions?
- Were the alternatives appropriate?
- How can you improve this?

Summary

- Teaching points relate primarily to the safety of the movements, and then to their effectiveness.
- Teaching position varies so that the instructor can see, and be seen by, all participants in the group at all times.
- Appropriate group organisation determines an effective teaching position.
- Explanations should be clear and precise and employ user-friendly language.
- The personal performance of the instructor should be strong, precise and correct.
- The voice of the instructor should be clear, audible and well-paced.
- The observational skills of the instructor should be excellent.
- Feedback should be clear and relevant to ensure the session is safe and effective.
- Feedback should be positive to motivate, encourage and increase participants' self-confidence.
- Alternatives and adaptations should be appropriate for a variety of postnatal problems and varying fitness levels.
- Self-evaluation assists professional development.
- Content and structure should be analysed for safety, effectiveness and enjoyment.
- Teaching elements should be considered in detail.
- Areas for improvement should be identified and changes instigated.

Abdominal and back care

Getting in and out of bed

| **Fig. A.1** | **Getting in and out of bed** |

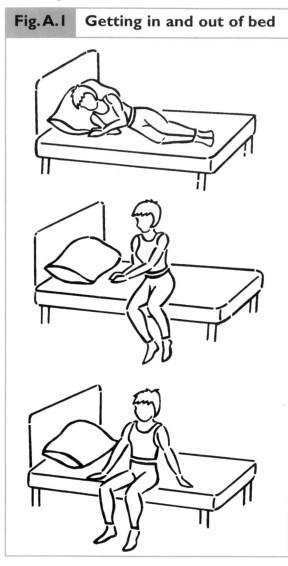

- Sit on the edge of the bed with your feet flat on the floor.
- Lie down on your side, draw navel to spine and lift your legs on to the bed.
- Moving the whole body, gently turn over on to your back keeping your knees and feet together.
- Reverse the process when getting out of bed.
- Avoid coming straight to a sitting position from lying down as this causes extreme stress to the abdominal muscles and the back.

Sitting up/getting out of the bath

If possible, roll on to your side as before, but if space is limited it is essential to draw navel through to spine to protect the abdominal muscles and back.

Standing whilst holding baby

When standing with baby on one shoulder, there may be a tendency to lean slightly backwards to keep the baby in position – particularly when it is very small and has no head control. If this is practised for long periods at a time the lumbar spine becomes stressed in this overextended position, which may induce backache. Be sure to stand in correct postural alignment, with the spine in neutral and the abdominal muscles lightly drawn in. Straddling the baby across one hip causes twisting in the pelvis and uneven pressure on the symphysis pubis and sacroiliac joints. Keeping the hips in line does not provide as much support for the baby but is much safer for the pelvis.

Fig. A.2 — Correct standing posture while holding baby

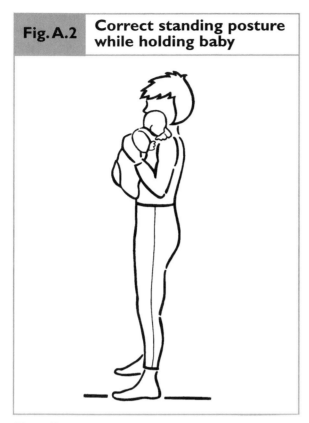

Fig. A.3 — Correct feeding posture

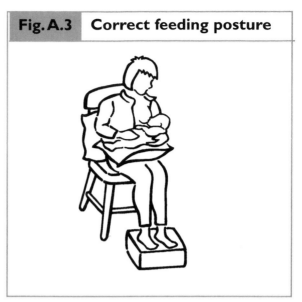

Maintaining correct seated posture may be extremely hard, particularly if you are finding breastfeeding difficult. A poor position may be held for some time if baby has problems latching on to the breast as it is feared that changing the position may disrupt the feed. Try to avoid this if possible.

Feeding posture

Whether you are breast- or bottle-feeding, the seated position you adopt is just as important as standing, as many hours may be spent there! Sitting in a slumped, bent position will cause additional back- and neck-ache. The following guidelines should be observed:

- Select a chair on which you can adopt an upright position – a very soft, bucket-shaped seat is not appropriate.
- Sit as far back into the chair as you can.
- Place cushions in the small of the back and sit tall.
- Put your feet on a footstool or pile of books to raise the height of your knees.
- Place your baby on a pillow on your lap to bring him closer to you.

Fig. A.4 — Bending and lifting

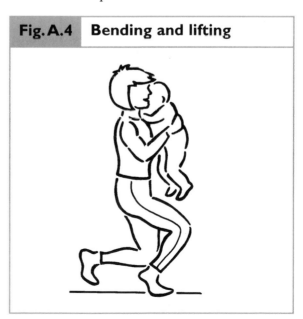

Bending down

- Use a wide base, with spine in neutral.
- Draw navel to spine and bend the knees, using the large muscles of the legs to lower you down.
- Keep the knees aligned over the ankles.
- Reverse the procedure to stand up.

Lifting

- Bend down, as above, as close as possible to the baby.
- Draw in the abdominal muscles.
- Bring the baby in close to you as you stand up.
- Use the strength of your legs to lift you.
- Avoid lifting heavy objects.

Fig. A.5	Changing baby

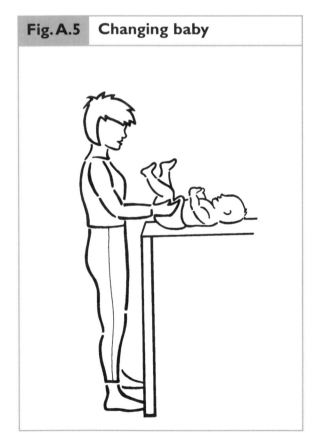

Changing baby

- Use a work surface that is at a correct height to prevent stooping.
- You may prefer to kneel next to the bed, although this may become very demanding on the knees.
- Position all your equipment in front or to your side to prevent twisting behind you.

Carrying baby

If carrying baby for any length of time it is much better to use a baby sling worn at the front and positioned as high as possible to avoid leaning back. When carrying shopping try to distribute the weight evenly between the bags and be sure to draw in the abdominal muscles to support the back. Alternatively, use a backpack.

Bathing baby

Lifting and lowering a heavy baby-bath full of water should be avoided at all costs. Choose a bath that rests over the main bath so you can fill and empty it in situ, and kneel alongside to bath the baby. Alternatively, use the bathroom handbasin when the baby is small.

Transitions between exercises

Whilst care and attention is given to the correct technique of the exercises themselves, the transitions between exercises also need clear guidelines.

Getting down to the floor

Bend the knees and use the large muscles in the legs to lower one knee to the floor. Maintain navel to spine and keep the knee aligned over the front ankle as you lower. Bring the other knee down and move onto hands and knees. Keeping knees and feet together, draw navel to spine and lower the buttocks to the floor, turning sideways into a seated position.

Moving from a seated position to supine lying

Always lie on your side first before moving onto your back. Keep the knees and feet together with navel to spine and turn the whole body over at the same time. Rolling the legs before the upper body will twist the lower back and pull on the oblique muscles.

Fig. A.6	**Safe transition to lying on the back**

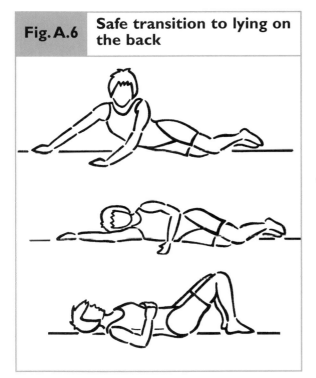

Returning from supine lying to a seated position

Place the knees and feet together, draw navel to spine and turn the whole body to the side at the same time. Use your arms to push you up to sitting.

Standing up

Via side lying, draw navel to spine and push up onto hands and knees. Walk the hands up the thighs to kneel up, draw navel to spine and bring one leg through in front and place the foot on the floor. Use a forward travelling motion to lift the body up to standing, rather than pushing down on the front thigh.

Rate of perceived exertion

This is a subjective method of assessing how hard you are working by rating the degree of physical exertion you feel. This is measured against the scale below for a reading between 0 and 10.

(Adapted from the revised Borg scale.)

Scale of perceived exertion

No exertion at all	0
Just perceptible	1
Extremely light	2
Very light	3
Light	4
Moderate	6
Hard	7
Very hard	8
Extremely hard	9
Maximum exertion	10

GLOSSARY

Abductors – gluteus medius and minimus muscles, covering the hip and pelvis, often referred to as the outer thigh muscles.

Acetabulum – cup-shaped socket which receives the head of the femur.

Actin – protein responsible for muscular contraction.

Adductors – the muscles of the inner thigh.

Amenorrhoea – cessation of menstruation.

Aponeurosis (abdominal) – a sheetlike, tendinous expansion connecting the abdominal musculature to the linea alba.

ASIS – anterior superior iliac spines – bony points at the front of the iliac crest.

Biceps – the muscles at the front of the upper arm.

Carpal tunnel syndrome – a condition associated with water retention where compression of the median nerve in the wrist causes tingling and numbness in the thumb, index and middle fingers.

Coccyx – four fused vertebrae joined to the sacrum, often referred to as the tail bone.

Cervical vertebrae – seven vertebrae in the upper back and neck.

Collagen – the main component of connective tissue.

Colostrum – a yellowish fluid produced by the breasts during pregnancy and the first few days after delivery.

Concentric contraction – the muscle shortens as it contracts.

Connective tissue – binds together and supports body structures (tendons, ligaments, cartilage, fascia, etc.).

Corpus luteum – the outer covering of the ovarian follicle, left behind after ovulation.

Decidua – the lining of the pregnant uterus.

Deltoids – the muscles covering the top of the shoulders.

Developmental stretching – stretching to increase the range of movement.

Diaphragm – the muscular partition between the abdominal and thoracic cavities.

Doming – a bulge in the abdominal wall occuring during contraction of rectus abdominis when the muscles are still separated.

Double pinning – a practice used in resistance training to limit the range of movement to ensure safety.

Embolus (air) – air entering the circulation and causing an obstruction.

Eccentric contraction – the muscle lengthens as it contracts.

Facet joints – the joining of the articular processes of two adjacent vertebrae.

Fascia – connective tissue separating muscle layers and encasing them in a sheath.

Femur – the thigh bone.

FITT – Frequency, Intensity, Time and Type – the methods used to increase fitness.

Fixator muscle – the muscle which stabilises the joint to prevent unnecessary movements while the prime mover is contracting.

Flexibility – movement of a joint beyond its natural range.

Gastrocnemius – the large muscle in the calf.

Gluteals – a group of muscles which cover the hip joint and much of the pelvis.

Gluteus medius/Gluteus minimus – a group of muscles attaching into the side and back of the pelvis, known collectively as the abductors.

Haemorrhoids – varicose veins of the anus.

Hamstrings – the muscles at the back of the thigh.

Hip flexors – the muscles connecting the lower spine and pelvis to the top of the femur.

Hyperextension – over-extending a joint (locking out).

Ileum – the wing-shaped part of the pelvis.

Iliopsoas – group of muscles referred to as the hip flexors.

Intra-abdominal pressure – pressure created by the synchronised contraction of transversus abdominis, diaphragm and pelvic floor to provide spinal support.

Ischial tuberosities – the sitting bones.

Ischium – the thick, lower part of the pelvis leading down to the ischial tuberosities.

Isometric – muscular contraction where the muscle stays the same length (static contraction).

Isotonic – muscular contraction where the muscle changes length (concentric or eccentric).

Kyphosis – exaggerated backward curvature of the thoracic spine.

Lactation – period of time relating to milk production.

Latissimus dorsi – the broad muscle in the middle and lower back.

Levator ani – the deep muscles of the pelvic floor.

Ligaments – connective tissue supporting the joints and organs.

Linea alba – a tendinous band situated down the mid-line of the abdomen, formed by the joining of the aponeurosis of the abdominal muscles.

Lithotomy (position) – where the legs are lifted into stirrups whilst lying supine – often used for perineal repair.

Lordosis – exaggerated forward curvature of the lumbar or cervical spine.

Lumbar vertebrae – five vertebrae of the lower back.

Maintenance stretching – stretches to maintain range of movement, normally of short duration hold.

Mastitis – an inflammation of the breast when milk is not emptied as quickly as it is produced.

Multifidus – a deep spinal muscle activated with transversus abdominis to provide core stabilisation.

Mobility – movement of a joint within its natural range.

Myosin – a protein responsible for muscular contraction (with actin).

Neutral spine – the natural, correct alignment of the spine which allows the body systems to function at their optimum.

Oestrogen – a female hormone, essential for the menstrual cycle, produced in large quantities during pregnancy when it is associated with the growth of the baby.

Obliques – two layers of abdominal muscle, the internal and external obliques, which are responsible for flexion and rotation of the trunk.

Overload – placing greater demands on the body than it is accustomed to.

Patella – the knee cap.

Pectoral muscles – the muscles of the chest.

Perineum – the area between the anus and the vagina.

Piriformis – a deep external rotator of the hip.

Prime mover – the key muscles responsible for joint action.

Principles of training – Frequency, Intensity, Time and Type – the method used to improve fitness.

Prolactin – the hormone responsible for stimulating milk production.

Prolapse – bulging of the bladder or rectum into the wall of the vagina or the descent of the uterus into the vagina.

Progesterone – a female hormone, essential to the menstrual cycle, produced in large quantities during pregnancy when it is responsible for relaxing smooth muscle tissue.

Prone – front lying.

Proprioception – the body's sense of position as a response from stimuli.

Pudendal nerve – responsible for activating the pelvic floor muscles.

Pubis – bone stituated at the front of the pelvis.

Q angle – the angle of the femur from the hips to the knee.

Quadriceps – a group of muscles at the front of the thigh.

Raphe – the mid-line where two symmetrical parts unite, i.e. linea alba.

Rec check – procedure for checking the abdominal muscles for separation before gravity-resisted exercises commence.

Rectus abdominis – the most superficial of the abdominal muscles which runs in two bands down the centre of the abdomen and undergoes tremendous stretching and separation during pregnancy.

Relaxin – a hormone produced in larger amounts during pregnancy to allow the pelvis to widen for delivery. Reduces stability of all joints.

Sacroiliac joints – two joints at the back of the pelvis formed by the unity of the ileum with the sacrum.

Sacrum – triangular-shaped bone made up of five fused vertebrae.

Sarcomere – the contractile unit of the muscle.

Sciatica – pain in the buttock which may radiate down the back of the leg.

Soleus – muscle in the lower calf.

Supine – back lying.

Symphysis pubis – the joint at the front of the pelvis joining the two pubic bones together.

Thoracic spine – the 12 vertebrae in the mid-section of the back.

Training effect – physiological adaptations of the body as a result of overload.

Transversus abdominis – the deepest abdominal muscle, responsible for compression of the abdominal wall and lumbar spine stabilisation.

Trapezius – triangular-shaped muscle in the neck and upper back.

Triceps – the muscles at the back of the upper arm.

Umbilicus – the navel.

Valsalva manoeuvre – the action of breath holding to increase intra-thoracic pressure as used by weight lifters.

Varicose veins – swollen veins with ineffective valves which are unable to close and secure one-way flow of blood.

Vastus medialis – a muscle of the quadriceps group specifically responsible for the last 15 degrees of knee extension.

Venous return – the flow of blood back to the heart.

REFERENCES

Bani, D. (1997). 'Relaxin: A Pleiotropic Hormone'. *General Pharmacology* 28(1): 13–22.

Blackburn, S. (2003). *Maternal, Fetal and Neonatal Physiology – A Clinical Perspective* Saunders.

Boissonault, J. (1998). 'The incidence of diastasis recti abdominis during the childbearing year'. *Physical Therapy* 68(7): 1082–1086.

Charelli, P. and Campbell, E. (1997). 'Incontinence during pregnancy: Prevalence and opportunities for continence promotion'. *Australian/New Zealand Journal of Obstetrics and Gynaecology* 37(1): 66–73.

Clapp, J.F. (1998). *Exercising through your pregnancy* Human Kinetics.

Cunningham, F.G., Macdonald P.C., Gant N.F., Gilstrap L.C., Harkins G.D.V., Clark S.L. Eds 1997. *Williams Obstetrics* (20th ed.) Stamford, CT: Appleton and Large 533–546.

Dewey, K.G., Lovelady, C.A., Nommsen-Rivers, L.A., McCrory, M.A. Lonerdal, B. (1994). 'A randomised study of the effects of aerobic exercise by lactating women on breast milk volume and composition'. *New England Journal of Medicine* 330: 449–453.

Drinkwater, B.L. and Chestnut, C.H. (1991). 'Bone density changes during pregnancy and lactation in active women'. *Bone Mineral* 14: 153–160.

Hodges, P.W. (1999). 'Is there a role for transversus abdominis in lumbo-pelvic stability?' *Manual Therapy* 4(2): 74–86.

Johnson, V.Y. (2001). 'How the principles of exercise physiology influence pelvic floor muscle training'. *Journal of WOCN* 3: 150–155.

Jozwik, M. and Jozwik, M. (1998). 'The physiological basis of pelvic floor exercises in the treatment of stress urinary incontinence'. *British Journal of Obstetrics and Gynaecology* 105: 1046–1051.

Kendall, F.P., McCreary, E.K. and Provance, P.G. (1993). *PG Muscles, Testing and Function*, 4th ed; Baltimore: Williams & Wilkins.

Kessel, K.V., Reed, S., Newton, K., Meier, A. and Lentz, G. (2001). 'The second stage of labour and stress urinary incontinence'. *American Journal of Obstetrics and Gynaecology* 184: 1571–1575.

King, J.K. and Freeman, R.M. (1998). 'Is antenatal bladder neck mobility a risk factor for postpartum stress incontinence?' *British Journal of Obstetrics and Gynaecology* 105: 1300–1307.

Lawrence, D. (1998). *The Complete Guide to Exercise in Water.* A&C Black.

Marshall, K., Totterdal, D., McConnell, V., Walsh, D.M. & Whelan, M. (1996) 'Urinary incontinence and constipation during pregnancy and after childbirth'. *Physiotherapy* 82(2): 98–103.

Morkved, S. and Bo, K. (1996). 'The effect of postnatal exercises to strengthen the pelvic floor muscles'. *Acta Obstet Gynaecol Scand* 75: 382–385.

Morkved, S. and Bo, K. (2000). 'Effect of postpartum pelvic floor muscle training in prevention and treatment of urinary incontinence'. *British Journal of Obstetrics and Gynaecology* 107: 1022–1028.

Norris, C. (2000) *Back Stability*, Human Kinetics.

Otis, C. and Goldingay, R. (2000). *The Athletic*

Woman's Survival Guide, Human Kinetics.

Quinn, T.J. and Carey, G.B. (1997). 'Is breast composition in lactating women altered by exercise intensity or diet?' *Medicine and Science in Sports and Exercise* 29–S4.

Richardson, C.A. and Jull, G.A. (1995). 'Muscle control – pain control. What exercises would you prescribe?' *Manual Therapy* 1: 2–10.

Sapsford, R.R., Markwell, S.J. and Clarke, B. (1998). 'The relationship between urethral pressure and abdominal muscle activity'. *Australian Continence Journal* 4: 102–104.

Sapsford, R.R., Hodges, P.W., Richardson, C.A., Cooper, D.H., Markwell, S.J. and Jull, G.A. (2001). 'Co-activation of the abdominal and pelvic floor muscles during voluntary exercises'. *Neurourology and Urodynamics* 20: 31–42.

Snooks, S.J., Swash, M., Mathers, S.E., Henry, M.M. (1990). 'Effect of vaginal delivery on the pelvic floor: a 5-year follow up'. *British Journal of Surgery* Vol 77: 1358–1360.

Vleeming, A., Stoeckart, R., Volkers, A.C.W., Snyders, C.J. (1990). 'Relation between form and function in the sacroiliac joint'. *Spine* 15: 130–32.

RECOMMENDED READING

Bean, Anita. *Complete Guide to Strength Training* (London: A & C Black, 1997).

Behnke, Robert S. *Kinetic Anatomy* (Human Kinetics 2001).

Byrne, Helene. *Exercise after Pregnancy* (Berkeley: Celestial Arts, 2001).

Calais-Germain, Blandine. *Anatomy of Movement* (Seattle: Eastland Press Inc., 1993).

Creager, Caroline. *Bounce Back into Shape after Baby*, (Berthould: Executive Therapy Ltd, 2001).

Creager, Caroline. *Therapeutic Exercises using Foam Rollers* (Berthoud Co: Executive Physical Therapy Inc 1996).

Creager, Caroline. *Therapeutic Exercises using Resistance Bands* (Berthoud Co: Executive Physical Therapy Inc 1998).

Lawrence, Debbie. *Complete Guide to Exercise to Music* (London: A & C Black, 1999).

Lawrence, Debbie. *Complete Guide to Exercise in Water* (London: A & C Black, 1998).

Mitchell, Laura. *Simple Relaxation* (London: John Murray, 1987)

Norris, Christopher M. *Back Stability* (Human Kinetics, 2000).

Robinson, Lynne et al. *Official Body Control Pilates Manual* (London: Macmillan 2000).

Sapsford, R., Bullock-Saxton, J., Markwell S.J. *Women's Health, A Textbook for physiotherapists* (London: Saunders, 1999).

USEFUL CONTACTS

The Association of Chartered Physiotherapists in Women's Health
Chartered Society of Physiotherapists
14 Bedford Row
London WC1R 4ED
tel 020 7306 6666
www.womensphysio.com

Baby Directory
tel 020 8742 8724
www.babydirectory.com
(Book of resources for parents and carers and useful advertising medium)

The Guild of Postnatal Exercise Teachers
tel 01453 884268
www.postnatalexercise.com
An organisation offering specialised teacher training courses for postnatal exercise

The National Childbirth Trust
Alexandra House
Oldham Terrace
Acton
London W3 6NH
tel 0870 444 8707
www.nct-online.org
www.nctpregnancyandbabycare.com

Parents Directory Publications
Needwood
West Lavant
Chichester
PO18 9AH
tel 01243 527605
(Book of resources for parents and carers and useful advertising medium for the London area)

Stability in Action
tel 01992 51129
info@stability-in-action.co.uk
An organisation offering teacher training courses on the use of the foam roller

Symphysis Pubis Dysfunction British Support Group
info@spd.uk.org
www.pregnancyandbabycare.com

INDEX